Handbook of
Treatment Planning in
Radiation Oncology

Handbook of Treatment Planning in Radiation Oncology

Gregory M. M. Videtic, MD, CM, FRCPC
Residency Program Director
Associate Professor of Medicine
Department of Radiation Oncology
Cleveland Clinic Foundation
Cleveland, Ohio

Andrew D. Vassil, MD
Resident Physician
Department of Radiation Oncology
Cleveland Clinic Foundation
Cleveland, Ohio

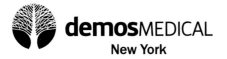

demosMEDICAL
New York

Acquisitions Editor: Richard Winters
Cover Design: Gary Ragaglia
Compositor: The Manila Typesetting Company
Printer: Odyssey Press Inc.

Visit our website at www.demosmedpub.com

Medicine is an ever-changing science. Research and clinical experience are continually expanding our knowledge, in particular our understanding of proper treatment and drug therapy. The authors, editors, and publisher have made every effort to ensure that all information in this book is in accordance with the state of knowledge at the time of production of the book. Nevertheless, the authors, editors, and publisher are not responsible for errors or omissions or for any consequences from application of the information in this book and make no warranty, express or implied, with respect to the contents of the publication. Every reader should examine carefully the package inserts accompanying each drug and should carefully check whether the dosage schedules mentioned therein or the contraindications stated by the manufacturer differ from the statements made in this book. Such examination is particularly important with drugs that are either rarely used or have been newly released on the market.

Library of Congress Cataloging-in-Publication Data

Handbook of treatment planning in radiation oncology / Gregory M.M. Videtic, Elie Elovic.
    p. ; cm.
  Includes bibliographical references and index.
  ISBN 978-1-933864-52-5 (alk. paper)
  1. Cancer--Radiotherapy--Handbooks, manuals, etc. 2. Cancer--Nursing--Handbooks, manuals, etc. I. Videtic, Gregory M. M. II. Elovic, Elie.
  [DNLM: 1. Neoplasms--radiotherapy--Handbooks. 2. Patient Care Planning--Handbooks. 3. Planning Techniques--Handbooks. 4. Radiotherapy--methods--Handbooks. QZ 39]
  RC271.R3H346 2011
  616.99'40642--dc22

                                                                    2010026507

Special discounts on bulk quantities of Demos Medical Publishing books are available to corporations, professional associations, pharmaceutical companies, health care organizations, and other qualifying groups. For details, please contact:
Special Sales Department
Demos Medical Publishing
11 W. 42nd Street, 15th Floor
New York, NY 10036
Phone: 800–532–8663 or 212–683–0072
Fax: 212–941–7842
E-mail: rsantana@demosmedpub.com

Made in the United States of America
10 11 12 13 14   5 4 3 2 1

Contents

Preface

The past decade has seen rapid changes in the field of radiation oncology, ranging from an increasing shift to "evidence-based" treatments, to a constantly expanding technological armamentarium. In this setting, the discipline's reference literature has also blossomed, with a large of variety of clinically-oriented textbooks and manuals becoming available to meet the needs both of busy trainees and clinicians engaged in the care of patients with cancer. For all that, radiation oncology remains a "technical" discipline, whose practice is gradually learned through experience, as it is handed down from "master to apprentice", typically in the familiar setting of the simulator room. Mindful of this, discussions with our residents at the Cleveland Clinic had suggested that there was a need for a focused pocket-sized handbook to act as quick resource for them as they carried out the steps during the planning and delivery of radiation therapy.

Handbook of Treatment Planning in Radiation Oncology is intended to be descriptive and not prescriptive. No treatment or equipment recommendations are being endorsed. Clinical stage descriptions employed the TNM definitions of the sixth edition of the *AJCC Cancer Staging Handbook*. In setting down the steps to follow in the treatment planning of an individual patient, there is no intent at providing comprehensive clinical algorithms for treatment decision-making. Rather, we have assumed that the indications for a particular therapy are known, and therefore, our focus is on a series of suggested steps to follow to successfully complete effective radiotherapy planning. Sections are organized by body site or system, whichever proved best for consistency in presenting the general principles of planning; for example, the chapter on thoracic malignancies includes esophageal cancers. We have also presented specialized topics such as palliative therapy and pediatrics. After referencing general planning requirements, each specific subsite within a given section then provides more specific details on approaches to radiotherapy planning. Although drawn from the wealth of clinical experience at our institution and the copious notes of the residents, numerous sources were referenced and reviewed to present the most up-to-date standards in our discipline. Recognizing that almost every component of radiation treatment can be considered an active area of investigation, we have deliberately limited our planning recommendations to what would be considered good and safe practice at this point. The detailed protocols available on-line from the Radiation Therapy Oncology Group (RTOG) were invaluable in providing structure and a model for outlining the steps in good radiotherapy planning. Ultimately, the practice of radiation oncology is an art—nothing can replace experience and many clinicians may debate the finer points in any given section. That said, guidelines provide structure and like a phrase book for a foreign language, they help put (sometimes) unknown or disparate terms together to form an intelligible concept. The competent professional will know when to move beyond these recommendations as required for individual patient care.

Handbook of Treatment Planning in Radiation Oncology represents the diligent efforts of our residents working under the guidance and mentorship of staff physicians. The quality of their chapters, their collaborative spirit, and their prompt response to feedback made the experience of editing their submissions a pleasure. The technical contributions of Nicole Pavelecky, CMD, staff dosimetrist, were invaluable in producing consistent images of high quality. Last but certainly not least, this project would not have been realized without the tireless dedication and outstanding contributions of Dr. Andrew Vassil, senior resident, and my coeditor.

Gregory M. M. Videtic, MD, CM, FRCPC
Andrew D. Vassil, MD

Contributors

All contributors of this text are affiliated with the Department of Radiation Oncology, Cleveland Clinic Foundation, Cleveland, Ohio.

Michael J. Burdick, MD

Samuel T. Chao, MD

Jay P. Ciezki, MD

John F. Greskovich, MD

Susan Guo, MD

Grant K. Hunter, MD

Justin J. Juliano, MD

Mohammad K. Khan, MD, PhD

Shlomo A. Koyfman, MD

Roger M. Macklis, MD

Anthony L. Magnelli, MS

Erin S. Murphy, MD

Nicole Pavelecky, CMD

Jerrold P. Saxton, MD

Lawrence J. Sheplan, MD

Kevin L. Stephans, MD

Abigail L. Stockham, MD

John H. Suh, MD

Rahul D. Tendulkar, MD

Andrew D. Vassil, MD

Gregory M. M. Videtic, MD, CM, FRCPC

Handbook of Treatment Planning in Radiation Oncology

1 General Physics Principles

Andrew D. Vassil, Nicole Pavelecky,
Anthony L. Magnelli, and Gregory M. M. Videtic

GENERAL PRINCIPLES

- Percent depth dose (PDD) is the ratio of absorbed dose (on the central axis) at a chosen depth to the absorbed dose at the reference point D_{max}.
- Normalizing dose refers to setting a desired dose point to which all other dose points are referred. For example, if one chooses to normalize to the D_{max} point, then all other points within the patient will receive a lesser dose (ie, the 100% isodose line is set to D_{max}).
- Isodose is the ratio of absorbed dose at a chosen point to the absorbed dose at a reference point (eg, the calculation point or isocenter).
- Depth dose (DD) is a function of
  - energy: as energy increases, DD increases
  - depth: as depth increases, DD decreases
  - source-surface distance (SSD): as SSD increases, DD decreases
  - field size: as field size increases, DD increases (due to increased scatter)
- D_{max} increases (moves deeper in the patient) as field size decreases. This is due to an increase in effective energy, as there is less collimator scatter, patient scatter, and transmission through the thicker portion of the flattening filter.
- "Hot spots" tend to increase in size as separation increases (eg, comparing plans on patients with a small vs large body mass index).
- Isodose lines shift as tissue electron density changes, and this is accounted for by "heterogeneity correction," for example, isodose lines move away from surface when beam goes through air and are brought toward surface when beam goes through bone.

- Source-surface distance (SSD) represents the distance between the radiation source and the treatment surface.
- Source-axis distance (SAD) represents the distance between the radiation source and the axis (isocenter) upon which the table, gantry, and collimator rotate.

TARGET VOLUMES

International Commission on Radiation Units & Measurements (ICRU) 50: "Prescribing, Recording, and Reporting Photon Beam Therapy"

- Gross tumor volume (GTV): gross palpable or visible/demonstrable extent and location of malignant growth.
- Clinical target volume (CTV): anatomical concept. Tissue volume that contains a GTV and/or a subclinical microscopic malignant disease that has to be eliminated.
- Planning target volume (PTV): geometrical concept. Defined to select appropriate beam sizes and beam arrangements, taking into consideration the net effect of all the possible geometrical variations and inaccuracies to ensure that the prescribed dose is actually absorbed in the CTV. Its size and shape not only depend on the CTV but also on the treatment technique used to compensate for the effects of organ and patient movement and inaccuracies in beam and patient setup.
- Treated volume: volume enclosed by an isodose surface (eg, 95% isodose), selected and specified as being appropriate in achieving the purpose of treatment. Ideally, treated volume would be identical to PTV but may also be considerably larger than PTV.
- Irradiated volume: tissue volume that receives a dose that is considered significant in relation to normal tissue tolerance. Dose should be expressed either in absolute values or relative to the specified dose to the PTV.
- Organs at risk (OAR): normal tissues whose radiation sensitivity may significantly influence treatment planning and/or prescribed dose.

TREATMENT PLANNING

Plan evaluation

- Review of the dose-volume histogram (DVH), maximum doses, minimum doses, mean doses, and isodose distribution on all axial images (high- and low-isodose lines) is essential when reviewing plans.
  - D percentage allows the analysis of a dose (D) that encompasses a percentage of a volume of interest (eg, D100, D90, and D80 represent the dose encompassing 100%, 90%, and 80% of a volume of interest, respectively).

- *V* percentage allows the analysis of a percent volume (*V*) that receives a particular dose (eg, V100, V90, and V80 represents the percent of a volume of interest that receives 100%, 90%, and 80% of the prescribed dose, respectively).

ICRU 50: "Prescribing, Recording, and Reporting Photon Beam Therapy" Recommendations for Reporting Dose

- ICRU reference point
  - Dose at the point should be clinically relevant and representative of the dose throughout PTV.
  - The point should be easy to define in a clear and unambiguous way.
  - The point should be selected where the dose can be accurately determined (physical accuracy).
  - The point should be selected in a region where there is no steep dose gradient.
  - The point should be located at the center of the PTV and, when possible, at the intersection of the beam axes.
  - The dose at the ICRU reference point is the ICRU reference dose.
- Dose at/near center of PTV, maximum dose to PTV, and minimum dose to PTV should always be reported.
- Maximum dose: highest dose in PTV. A volume is considered clinically meaningful if its minimum diameter exceeds 15 mm; however, if it occurs in a small organ (eg, the eye, optic nerve, larynx), a dimension smaller than 15 mm has to be considered.
- Minimum dose: lowest dose in PTV. In contrast to maximum dose, no volume limit is recommended.
- Hot spots: volume outside the PTV that receives dose larger than 100% of the specified PTV dose. In general, a hot spot is considered significant only if the minimum diameter exceeds 15 mm; however, if it occurs in a small organ (eg, the eye, optic nerve, larynx), a dimension smaller than 15 mm has to be considered.

ICRU 62 "Prescribing, Recording, and Reporting Photon Beam Therapy (Supplement to ICRU Report 50)"

Global concept and definition of PTV is not changed, but the definition is supplemented.

- Internal margin (IM): variations in size, shape, and position of the CTV relative to anatomic reference points (eg, filling of bladder, movements of respiration). The internal variations are physiological ones and result in change in site, size, and shape of the CTV.

- Internal target volume (ITV): volume encompassing the CTV and IM (ITV = CTV + IM).
- Setup margin (SM): uncertainties in patient positioning and alignment of therapeutic beams during treatment planning and through all treatment sessions. The uncertainities may vary with selection of beam geometries and may depend on variations in patient positioning, mechanical uncertainities of the equipment (eg, sagging of gantry, collimators, or couch), dosimetric uncertainities, transfer setup errors from simulator to treatment unit, and human factors. These may vary from center to center and from machine to machine.
- Planning target volume (PTV) = CTV + IM + SM. The penumbra of the beam(s) is not considered when delineating the PTV. However, when selecting beam sizes, the width of the penumbra has to be taken into account and the beam size adjusted accordingly.
- A dose variation between 7% and −5% is generally accepted.
- Conformity index: treated volume/PTV. It is implied that treated volume completely encompasses the PTV.
- Organs at risk volumes:
  - Organs at risk (OAR): normal tissues whose radiation sensitivity may significantly influence treatment planning and/or prescribed dose.
  - Planning organ at risk volume (PRV): analogous to PTV for OAR. PRV = OAR + IM + SM.

- Dosing
  - Biologically effective dose (BED) calculations are based on the linear quadratic model of radiation effect.
  - BED equations are used to compare various fractionation schemes for their potential effects on early and late responding tissues. Depending on the clinical scenario, BED for late effects drives the choice of dose and fraction.
  - α/β ratio represents the inherent sensitivity to fractionation.
  - An α/β ratio of 3 is used for late responding tissues and 10 for early responding tissues (and most epithelial tumors).
  - BED = $(nd) \times [1 + (d/\{\alpha/\beta\})]$, where n is the number of fractions and d is dose per fraction
    - 78 Gy/2 Gy/fx, 39 fx, 5 fx per week.
      Early effects: $(39 \times 2) \times [1 + (2/10)] = 93.6 \text{ Gy}_{10}$
      Late effects: $(39 \times 2) \times [1 + (2/3)] = 130 \text{ Gy}_3$
    - 70 Gy/2.5 Gy/fx, 28 fx, 5 fx per week.
      Early effects: $(28 \times 2.5) \times [1 + (2.5/10)] = 87.5 \text{ Gy}_{10}$
      Late effects: $(28 \times 2.5) \times [1 + (2.5/3)] = 128 \text{ Gy}_3$

TABLE 1.1 Percentage of Normal Bone Marrow Irradiated Using Standard Radiation Ports

Site	Marrow Volume at Risk
Skull (not including mandible)	12%
Upper limb girdle (unilateral, including humeral head, scapulae, clavicle)	4%
Sternum	2%
Ribs (all)	8%
Ribs (hemithorax)	4%
Cervical vertebrae (all)	3%
Thoracic vertebrae (all)	14%
Lumbar vertebrae (all)	11%
Sacrum	14%
Pelvis	26%
Mantle field	25%
Upper para-aortic lymph nodes	45%

Data were derived from Ellis RE, *Physics in Medicine and Biology*, Vol. 5, 1961.

- Percentage of normal bone marrow irradiated using standard radiation ports (Table 1.1) (1).

- Block margins versus dosimetric margins
  - Using "block margins," the secondary collimator [cerrobend block or multileaf collimator (MLC)] expands circumferentially beyond the target by a fixed distance ("block margin") as seen by a beam's eye view.
  - Using "dosimetric margins," dose is prescribed to a chosen circumferential expansion around a defined volume.

- Wedges
  - Wedges are tissue compensators.
  - They are used to alter isodose distribution to a defined angle (Figure 1.1).
  - Physical wedges are placed in the beam path to attenuate the beam.
  - Dynamic wedge is the movement of the primary collimator while the beam is on to vary intensity across the field.
- A wedged pair is useful for superficial lesions (Figure 1.2).
  - A pair set of coplaner beams is designed with wedging designed to produce a more homogenous isodose distribution.

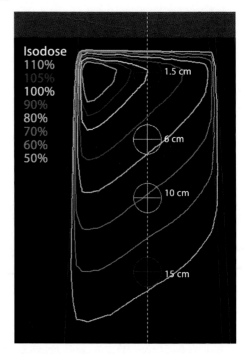

FIGURE 1.1 Isodose distribution in a tissue equivalent phantom using a 6-MV photon field with a 45° physical wedge (10 × 10 cm field size, 100 SAD, isocenter at D_{max}).

■ The "heal" of the wedge is placed inward. Wedge angle = 90 − (hinge angle/2); however, determining the optimal wedge angle may require multiple planning trials.

■ Field matching
　■ At an electron/photon beam interface, the hot spot is just inside the photon beam (due to bulging out of the electron field isodose distribution) (see Figure 1.3).
　■ Match junction may be shifted every 8 to 10 Gy by 0.5 to 1 cm to minimize cumulative overlap, also known as "feathering the junction."
　■ The light field represents the photon 50% isodose line.

■ Blocking
　■ Field blocking is accomplished through cerrobend blocks and/or multileaf collimators.
　■ There is ~ 7%-10% transmission through a half-beam cut block, 4%-7% through a corner block, and 1%-2% through the primary collimator (varies due to differences in scatter).
　■ Cerrobend is made of bismuth, tin, lead, and cadmium.

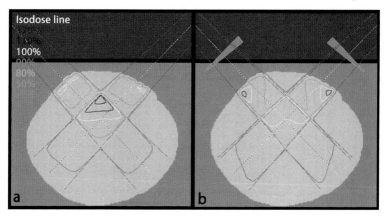

FIGURE 1.2 Isodose distribution in a simulated curved tissue equivalent phantom using a pair of 6-MV photon fields (10 × 10 cm field size, 100 SAD) (a) showing the influence of 45° physical wedges on isodose distribution (b). The only difference between the figures is the presence of the wedges.

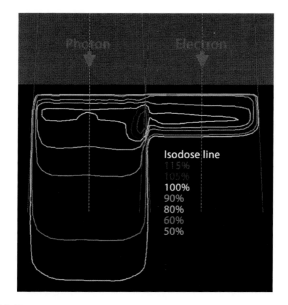

FIGURE 1.3 Example of photon-electron field match in a tissue equivalent phantom. A 6-MV photon field (10 × 10 cm field size, 100 SAD, isocenter at D_{max}) and a 9-MV photon field (10 × 10 cm cone, 100 SAD, isocenter at surface) were normalized to D_{max}.

- A half value layer (HVL) is the amount of material that allows 50% transmission.
- HVL increases due to "beam hardening" (ie, attenuation of lower energy beams).
- Amount remaining (transmission): 10% transmission through 3.3 HVL, 1% through 6.6 HVL, and 0.1% after 10 HVL

- Bolus
  - Bolus material is used to increase surface dose through beam interaction before a beam enters a patient.
  - Its electron density should be similar to that of tissue.
  - Synthetic materials are available, and alternatives include paraffin wax, towels soaked in water, ultrasound gel in a bag.

SELECTED TECHNICAL FACTS

- Beam characteristics (Table 1.2)
- Photon and electron beam central axis PDD curves for selected energies (Figure 1.4a and b)
- Isodose distributions of various PA and AP/PA photon fields (Figures 1.5 and 1.6)
- Isodose distributions of en-face electron fields (Figure 1.7)
- Interactions of photons with matter:
  - Coherent scattering: only important in diagnostic x rays (energy is unchanged, only direction has changed)
  - Photoelectric effect: photon in, electron and characteristic x rays out (probability proportional to Z^3/E^3)
  - Compton scattering/incoherent scatter: photon in, electron and photon out (probability proportional to $1/E$, independent of Z, Compton component begins to dominate at energies of ~200 KV)

TABLE 1.2 Selected Beam Characteristics

Photons	Electrons
^{60}Co: D_{max} = 0.5 cm, attenuation ~5%/cm	MeV/5 = D_{max} (cm)
4 MV: D_{max} = 1.0 cm	MeV/4 = 90% IDL
6 MV: D_{max} = 1.5 cm, attenuation ~4%/cm	MeV/3 = 80% IDL
10 MV: D_{max} = 2.5 cm	MeV/2.33 = 50% IDL
18 MV: D_{max} = 3.5 cm, attenuation ~3%/cm	MeV/2 = R_p

Abbreviations: ^{60}Co, Cobalt 60; IDL, isodole line; R_p, practical range.

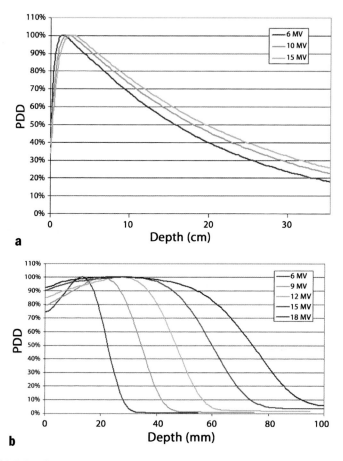

FIGURE 1.4 (a) Photon depth-dose curves, 10 × 10 cm field, 100 SSD. (b) Electron depth-dose curves, 10 × 10 cm electron cone, 100 SSD. Note: Surface dose decreases with increasing photon energy and increases with increasing electron energy.

- Pair production: photon in, electron and positron out (requires 1.02 MV threshold)
- Photodisintegration: photon in, neutron or proton out (also known as γ,*n* or γ,*p* reaction, requires ~ 7 MV threshold)

- Interactions of electrons with matter:
  - Inelastic collision with atomic nucleus: bremsstrahlung
  - Inelastic collision with atomic electrons: ionization or excitation

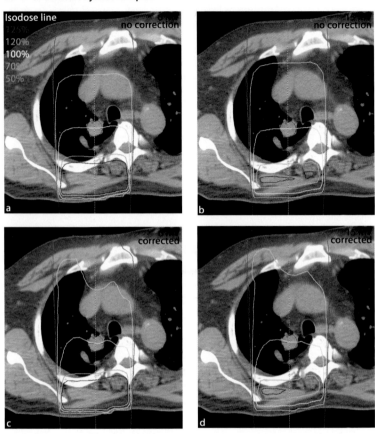

FIGURE 1.5 Posteroanterior beam, 10 × 10 cm fields, 100 SAD, dose normalized to isocenter placed at a 9-cm depth: (a) 6- and (b) 15-MV photons without heterogeneity correction; (c) 6- and (d) 15-MV photons with heterogeneity correction.

- Elastic collision with atomic nucleus
- Elastic collision with atomic electrons

■ Important characteristics of electron beams:
- Obliquity should be avoided with electron fields as surface dose increases, and penetration decreases, and D_{max} moves toward the surface secondary to scatter.
- Isodose line "bulging" (Figure 1.7):
  - Low-isodose lines bulge out for both high- and low-energy electrons.

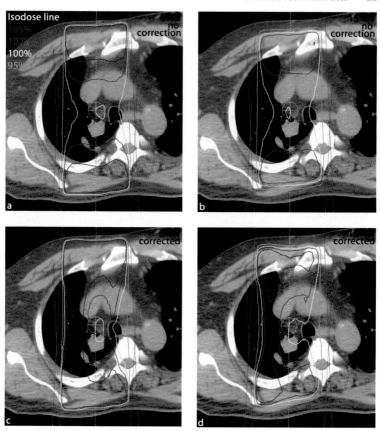

FIGURE 1.6 Anteroposterior/posteroanterior beams, 10 × 10 cm fields, 100 SAD, dose normalized to midplane: (a) 6- and (b) 15-MV photons without heterogeneity correction; (c) 6- and 15-MV (d) photons with heterogeneity correction.

- High-isodose lines constrict for high-energy electrons (not for low-energy electrons).
- Surface dose increases with increasing electron energy due to increased side-scatter.
- X-ray contamination is greater for high-energy electron beams and highest at the beams central axis (mainly due to bremsstrahlung interactions with the scattering foil).
- The minimum field diameter for an electron beam should be energy/2 (to allow for adequate scatter for dose buildup).
- DD decreases as field size decreases.

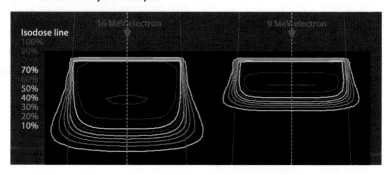

FIGURE 1.7 Isodose distributions of 16- and 9-MV electrons are compared to emphasize greater constriction of high-isodose lines when using high-energy electron beams.

SELECTED BRACHYTHERAPY FACTS

- Isotope properties (Table 1.3).
- Principles of decay
  - Decay constant (λ): fraction decaying/unit time = 0.693/half-life
  - Half-life = 0.693/decay constant

TABLE 1.3 Isotopes

Radionuclide	Decay Mode	Beta Energy
Pd-103	Electron capture	None
I-125	Electron capture	None
Ir-192	Gamma	240-670 KV
Au-198	Gamma	0.96 MV (max)
Cs-137	Gamma	0.514-1.17 MV
Ra-226	Gamma	0.017-3.26 MV
Co-60	Gamma	313 KV (max)
I-131	Beta	791 KV (max); 180 KV (avg)
Sr-89	Beta	1.46 MV (max); 583 KV (avg)
P-32	Beta	1.7 MV (max); 695 KV (avg)
Y-90	Beta	2.282 MV (max); 937 KV (avg)
Ru-106	Beta	3.54 MV (max)
Sm-153	Mixed	233 KV (avg)

Abbreviations: avg, Average; Au, gold; Co, cobalt; Cs, cesium; I, iodine; Ir, iridium; P, phosphorus; Pd, palladium; Ra, radium; Ru, ruthenium; Sm, samarium; Sr, strontium; Y, yttrium.

Exposure rate constant in R cm^2/h mCi except for radium and radon (R cm^2/h mg).

- Current activity or number of atoms = (initial activity or number of atoms) $\times e^{-\lambda \times time}$
- Rules of thumb regarding decay:
  - Amount remaining: 10% remains after 3.3 half-lives, 1% after 6.6 half-lives, 0.1% after 10 half-lives
  - Cs-137: ~2.3% decay per year
  - Co-60: ~1% decay per month
  - I-125 and Ir-192: ~1% decay per day
  - Pd-103: ~4% decay per day

ICRU 38 "Dose and Volume Specification for Reporting Intracavitary Therapy in Gynecology"

- Low dose rates (LDR), between 0.4 and 2 Gy/h; high dose rates (HDR), >12 Gy/h
- Bladder reference point:
  - Foley catheter is inserted and the balloon filled with 7-cm^3 radio-opaque contrast fluid. Tension is applied to bring catheter against the urethra.
  - Lateral radiograph: posterior surface of the balloon on an AP line drawn through the center of the balloon
  - AP radiograph: center of the balloon

Gamma Energy	Half-Life	Exposure Rate Constant*	Lead HVL, mm
21 KV (avg)	17 d	1.48	0.008
28 KV (avg)	60.2 d	1.46	0.025
380 KV (avg)	74.2 d	4.69	2.5
412 KV	2.7 d	2.38	2.5
662 KV (max)	30 y	3.26	5.5
830 KV (avg)	1622 y	8.25	12
1.25 MV (avg)	5.26 y	13.07	11
80-637 KV	8 d	2.2	3
–	50.5 d	–	–
–	14.3 d	–	0.1
–	64 h	–	–
–	366 d	–	–
103 KV (avg)	1.93 d		

- Rectal reference point:
  - Visualize posterior vaginal wall with opacification of the vaginal cavity with radio-opaque gauze used for packing.
  - Lateral radiograph: an AP line is drawn from the lower end of the intrauterine source (or the middle of the intravaginal source). Reference point is on this line, 5 mm behind posterior vaginal wall.
  - AP radiograph: the reference point is at the lower end of the intrauterine source (or the middle of the intravaginal source).

REFERENCE

1. Ellis RE. The distribution of active bone marrow in the adult. *Phys Med Biol* 1961;5:255-258.

2 Tools for Simulation and Treatment

Andrew D. Vassil and Gregory M. M. Videtic

TECHNIQUES IN POSITIONING AND IMMOBILIZATION

Thermoplastic mesh

- Thermoplastic mesh is a polymer that becomes soft and flexible when heated in a water bath, providing a customizable material for reproducible immobilization.
- Thermoplastic mesh is most commonly used for immobilizing the head but may be used at other sites such as the abdomen or extremities.
- Three-point masks (Figure 2.1a) are commonly used for brain and head and neck treatments.
- Bolus material may be held to the region of interest with the use of a swimmer's cap under a thermoplastic mesh mask (Figure 2.1b).

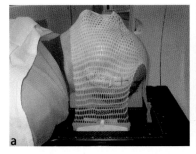 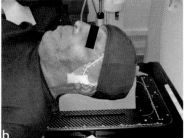

FIGURE 2.1 (a) Patient with a 3-point thermoplastic mask (points superior and lateral to head fixed to table). (b) Swimmer's cap used to hold tissue-equivalent bolus material to a region of interest.

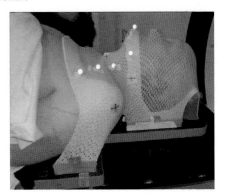

FIGURE 2.2 Patient with 5-point thermoplastic mask (points superior, lateral to head, and shoulders fixed to table).

- Five-point masks (Figure 2.2) provide additional immobilization of the shoulders and are particularly useful for stereotactic treatments.
- Body molds (Figure 2.3) may be created to aid in abdominal and pelvic treatments.

Cradle-type devices

- Molds occupying the space between the treatment table and the patient can be custom-made to provide a reproducible positioning system.
- Materials such as foam used in Alpha cradles and vacuum locking beads in airtight bags (eg, Elekta BodyFIX, Stockholm, Sweden). Patients are placed in the cradle, and vacuum suction is applied, locking the beads in place.
- Partial-body cradles are used for immobilization of a portion of the body, for example, an extremity (Figure 2.4a).

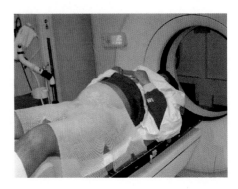

FIGURE 2.3 Thermoplastic body mold.

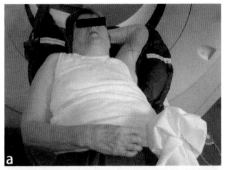

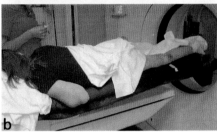

FIGURE 2.4 (a) Woman with sarcoma of the left arm, immobilized in a partial-body vacuum locking bag. (b) Woman with sarcoma of the left leg, immobilized prone in a full-body vacuum locking bag.

- Full-body cradle is used for stereotactic treatments and when immobilization at multiple points is desired (Figure 2.4b).

Modular systems

- Modular systems exist for custom immobilization of nearly every body site; an example is shown in Figure 2.5a and b.
- Custom adjustments can be made via modules to position the head, arms, chest, abdomen, pelvis, and legs.
- "Belly board" systems position the patient prone; a space exists for anterior displacement of abdominal contents (Figure 2.5c).

Stereotactic systems

- BodyFIX with total body cover sheet
  - Uses a full-body vacuum-locking (vac-loc) bag (BodyFIX) beneath the patient with a thin plastic sheet that covers the patient. The thin plastic sheet is attached to the vac-loc bag by an adhesive film at the edges. Vacuum suction is applied to remove air between the thin plastic sheet and the vac-loc bag to further limit the patient's motion (Figure 2.6).

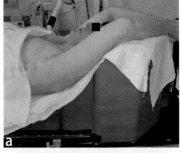

FIGURE 2.5 Modular positioning system for upper (a) and lower (b) body positioning. Also shown is a belly board for anterior displacement of bowel (c).

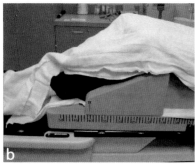

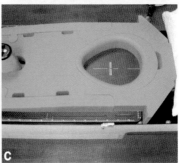

Breath control systems

- Abdominal compression
  - An adjustable paddle placed in the epigastric region or a belt placed at the level of the umbilicus is adjusted to restrict breathing to a tolerable level that minimizes target motion (Figure 2.7).
  - Choice of paddle or belt depends on target location; less interference occurs using a belt for patients with inferiorly located chest lesions.
- Breath control
  - Breath-holding techniques, for example, an active breathing control, often use valves to control airflow through a mouthpiece. The breath

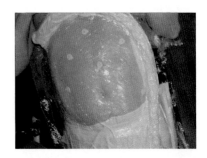

FIGURE 2.6 Patient positioned supine in a full-body vacuum locking bag. A vacuum-sealed total body cover sheet is covering the patient to provide additional immobilization. Adhesive attachments for infrared markers are present on the cover sheet.

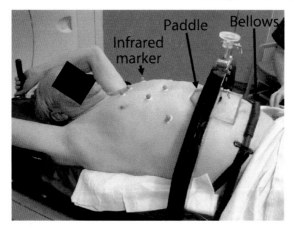

FIGURE 2.7 Patient positioned supine with arms above the head using a combined modular arm immobilization system and a full-body vacuum locking bag. Abdominal compression is applied with an adjustable paddle to restrict tumor motion. A bellows system is in place to track respiratory phase for 4D-CT. Infrared markers are part of the IGRT verification system for use at the time of treatment.

holding is conducted during simulation and replicated at the treatment machine.
- Chairs
  - Patients in distress who cannot lay flat or recline may, in emergency situations, be treated in the sitting position using a suitably designed chair providing stability and a reference system.

TECHNIQUES IN SIMULATION

- 2-Dimensional (fluoroscopy)
  - Fluoroscopy is used to position the patient based on disease, bony landmarks, and radiopaque wires placed by the physician.
  - Radiographs are made to include the entire treatment volume, from which custom blocks may be designed to avoid normal tissue.
- 3-Dimensional (CT)
  - Conventional CT images are acquired.
  - The isocenter is placed within the tumor volume (a least D_{max} from the surface).
  - Marks are placed on the patient for triangulation to the isocenter.
  - Shifts from this isocenter may be made at the time of treatment planning.

- Allows for planning based on 3D volumes, creation of beam's-eye-view, and highly conformal planning, both forward and inverse.
- 4-Dimensional (4D-CT)
    - Allows for visualization of target and organ motion.
    - Computed tomography image sets are acquired over consecutive breathing cycles. They are sorted for viewing by respiratory phase detected by a fiducial system and/or a device to record the respiratory cycle, for example, Varian (Palo Alto, CA) RPM and Philips (Andover, MA) abdominal bellows device (Figure 2.7).
- Contouring volumes
    - The advent of computer treatment planning systems using 3D and 4D imaging has allowed for physicians to create "volumes" that represent target and normal structures.
    - The Radiation Therapy Oncology Group (RTOG) has made numerous atlases available to aid in contouring volumes (http://208.251.169.72/atlases/contour.html).
    - Secondary image sets can be coregistered with simulation CT images to aid in volume localization (eg, MRI, PET, Magnetic Resonance Spectroscopy (MRS), and angiogram).
    - Maximal intensity projection (MIP) renders images from multiple phases to a display of maximal volume. For example, images generated from all phases of a respiratory cycle (from a 4D-CT) may be shown as one set to allow the physician to see structure location changes that will occur during respiration.

TECHNIQUES IN LOCALIZATION AT THE TIME OF TREATMENT DELIVERY

Gaiting

- Gaiting techniques coordinate the timing of radiation beam "on-time" with a desired target position, as determined by a reference fiducial system.
    - For example, beam-on within a selected phase of the respiratory cycle (eg, rest phase of exhalation)

Portal imaging

- Megavoltage radiographs may be taken prior to treatment delivery to confirm patient's positioning.
    - These are recommended to be conducted at least weekly
    - Orthogonal films (eg, AP and lateral) allow for corrections in patient's position.
    - Electronic (digital) portal imaging uses amorphous silicon to create digital portal films.

Image-guided radiation therapy (IGRT)

- Radiotherapy (RT) delivery where high precision was provided by requiring daily verification of setup prior to treatment, using target or other reference structures (eg, bone), defines IGRT.
- Ultrasound
  - May be referenced to simulation CT or ultrasound conducted at the time of simulation (Figure 2.8)
  - Non-ionizing method to locate target
  - Has issues of interuser variability (eg, the amount of pressure applied and the location where the transducer is placed)
  - Most commonly used to locate prostate and prostatic bed; more recently used to locate breast tumor bed
- In-room orthogonal radiographs
  - Mounted to gantry or in ceiling and floor
  - Radiography central axes intersect at the isocenter
  - Uses bony landmark or implanted fiducial markers as a reference point
  - Allows for intrafraction monitoring (ie, imaging while the therapeutic beam is turned on)
- Calypso beacon transponders
  - Radiofrequency transponders
    - Require implantation
    - Currently only used routinely for prostate radiotherapy (Figure 2.9)
  - Allow for triangulation and intrafraction tracking

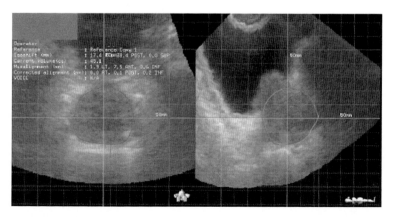

FIGURE 2.8 Transabdominal ultrasound in coronal and sagittal planes used for prostate localization for a patient receiving imaged-guided IMRT.

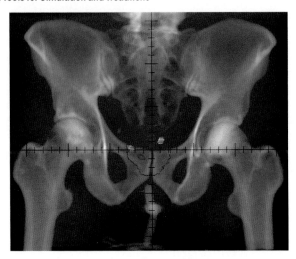

FIGURE 2.9 AP digitally reconstructed radiograph of a patient with implanted Calypso beacon transponders (green, yellow, and blue); the prostate is outlined in red. The patient also has an urethrogram study.

- Cone beam and helical imaging
    - Kilovoltage or MV imaging may be used to locate structures on the day of treatment (Figure 2.10). Alignment may be made to bone or soft tissue.
    - Kilovoltage radiography tube is mounted 90° to the gantry or in line with the gantry.
    - Megavoltage imaging using linear accelerator beam (may be degraded to KV energy to improve resolution). Translating the table during image acquisition provides helical imaging.

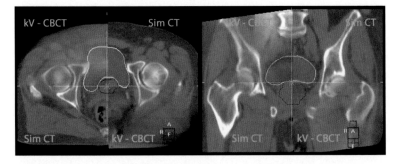

FIGURE 2.10 KV cone beam CT used for image-guided radiotherapy from of a patient with prostate cancer. Axial and coronal images are shown colocalized with the simulation CT.

- Volumetric information for understanding of positional errors in the x, y, z, roll, pitch, and yaw directions is given.
- CT on rails
  - Mobile diagnostic-type KV CT scanner in treatment vault.
  - CT translates over the patient on a rail system.
  - Allows for high-resolution, diagnostic-quality imaging.
- Doses from techniques that use ionizing radiation are in the range of 0.1 cGy for orthogonal KV systems and 1 to 10 cGy per fraction for KV and MV cone beam scans, depending on field size and amount of rotation.
- Treatment tables with 6° of motion freedom (x, y, z, roll, pitch, and yaw) have been developed to compensate for deviations in setup found with image-guided radiation therapy.
- Monitoring of external fiducial markers or light surface projections
  - Infrared markers placed on the patient may be monitored with in-room infrared cameras.

3 Central Nervous System Radiotherapy

Abigail L. Stockham, John H. Suh, and Samuel T. Chao

GENERAL PRINCIPLES

- General principles for simulation techniques, dose constraints, and planning principles apply to a range of intracranial tumors.
- Dose prescriptions are specific to a range of patient, tumor, and treatment factors relevant to the individual case.
- Postoperative radiotherapy is usually started 2 to 4 weeks after resections for malignant disease; benign resected tumors may be treated further from resection.

Localization, Immobilization, and Simulation

- CT simulation to delineate GTV, CTV, and PTV.
- The patient is positioned supine with arms at the sides.

- Immobilization is achieved with a thermoplastic mask. Head frame is usually used for single-fraction SRS.
- Use spiral CT to plan with 2- to 3-mm slice acquisition from the vertex through the mid-cervical spine. IV contrast for enhancing lesions may be used to delineate the tumor volume/resection cavity.
- MRI simulation may be used to avoid issues of coregistration.

Target Volumes and Organs of Interest Definition

- GTV: tumor volume or postoperative resection cavity appreciable on radiographic imaging, typically MRI.
- CTV: includes sites at risk for microscopic disease.
- PTV: allows for daily variation in setup and varies from institution to institution based on that institution's ability to reproduce treatment positions. Consider tighter margins when using image-guided radiation therapy.
- Regions of interest are identified and contoured (see Table 3.1).

Treatment Planning

Planning

- Treatment planning is optimized with MRI coregistration to assist in delineating edema with T2 and fluid attenuation and inversion recovery (FLAIR) images as well as to discern the presence or extent of T1-enhancing lesions.
- MRIs used in treatment planning should be obtained postoperatively within 48 hours to avoid ambiguity regarding residual tumor versus postoperative changes/blood. Timing of MRIs for treatment planning for benign processes is less critical.

Options

- Point calculations: primarily used in palliative treatment such as whole-brain EBRT (see Chapter 13).
- 3-D conformal radiotherapy: standard coplanar or noncoplanar 3D conformal fields are structured to optimize dose to target areas while minimizing dose to critical structures.
- IMRT: increasingly used to spare critical structures of the brain/spine for its ability to deliver a highly conformal dose to a target while respecting dose constraints to critical structures.
- Image-guided radiotherapy: used for lesions particularly close to critical structures (usually in the setting of IMRT) to ensure accurate daily setup.

TABLE 3.1 Maximum Point Doses for Fractionated Radiotherapy and SRS for Intracranial Structures of Interest

Structures of Interest	Maximum Point Dose, Gy	
	Fractionated Radiotherapy	SRS
Lenses	7	As low as possible
Retina	45–50	As low as possible
Optic nerves	55	8
Optic chiasm	56	8
Cochlea	55	8–9
Pituitary	45	As low as possible
Brainstem	60	12
Spinal cord	50	10

Abbreviation: SRS, stereotactic radiosurgery.

Critical Structures

The brain contains several structures considered to be "serial structures" emphasizing the importance of evaluating point doses in addition to volumetric doses (see Table 3.1).

Single Fraction SRS

Indications
- Benign and malignant brain tumors, vascular malformations, and functional disorders.
- Single-fraction SRS alone is most appropriate for well-circumscribed targets (≤4 cm in diameter; 0.3-0.5 cm from optic apparatus).
- Consider fractionated radiotherapy for tumors too large for SRS or abutting critical structures, especially optic nerve and chiasm.

SRS technique
- Intravenous line placed for midazolam sedation.
- Lidocaine injected at 4 locations on the scalp for frame placement.
- Image with MRI (1-mm slices) then CT. Coregister scans.
- Planning: Volume is T1 enhancing tumor or other anatomic structures for functional disorders.
- 6 to 10 mg dexamethasone IV 30 minutes before the procedure (consider continuing dexamethasone for 1-2 weeks postprocedure if concerned for edema).

SRS planning goals

■ The conformality index, the ratio of the prescription isodose volume divided by the tumor volume, should be ≤2. The homogeneity index, or the ratio of the maximum dose divided by the peripheral dose, should be ≤2.

■ PTV is enhancing lesion on T1 MRI with gadolinium. For very superficial lesions bolus may be used, held in place by a swimmer's cap.

GLIOMA—HIGH GRADE

Indications and Options for Treatment

■ Adjuvant therapy in the postoperative setting.
■ Definitive treatment in the inoperable setting.

Localization, Immobilization, Simulation for Fractionated RT/Fractionated Stereotactic RT (FSRT)

■ Per general principles.

Volumes, Dose, and Fractionation

■ Anaplastic astrocytoma
  ■ Volumes
    • GTV: postoperative T1-weighted MRI contrast enhancement or T2 signal change.
    • CTV: GTV + 1.5 to 2 cm
    • PTV: CTV + 0.3 to 0.5 cm
  ■ Dose and fractionation
    • 50.4 Gy/1.8 Gy/fx to initial field as above
    • Boost 9 Gy/1.8 Gy/fx to the postoperative contrast-enhancing tumor on T1-weighted MRI GTV with a 1.0 cm margin for CTV.
■ Anaplastic oligodendroglioma
  ■ Volumes
    • GTV: postoperative T2 MRI changes
    • CTV: GTV + 1.5 to 2 cm
    • PTV: CTV + 0.3 to 0.5 cm
  ■ Dose and fractionation
    • 50.4 Gy/1.8 Gy/fx to initial field as above
    • Boost 9 Gy/1.8 Gy/fx to postoperative contrast-enhancing tumor on T1-weighted MRI GTV with a 1.0-cm margin for CTV
■ Glioblastoma (see Figure 3.1)
  ■ Volumes
    • GTV: postoperative resection cavity, contrast enhancement, or edema on T2/FLAIR.

- CTV: GTV + 2 cm if edema on T2/FLAIR or 2.5 cm if no edema with respect for natural boundaries.
- PTV: CTV + 0.3 to 0.5 cm
- Dose and fractionation
  - 46 Gy/2 Gy/fx to T2/FLAIR change as above.
  - Boost 14 Gy/2 Gy/fx to the resection cavity or postoperative T1 contrast enhancement (GTV) with a 2.0-cm margin for CTV and 0.3 to 0.5 cm PTV.

Special Considerations
- Elderly patients or patients with poor performance status may be considered for altered fractionation, including:
  - 40 Gy/2.67 Gy/fx
  - 37.5 Gy/2.5 Gy/fx
  - 30 Gy/3 Gy/fx (as whole-brain RT)

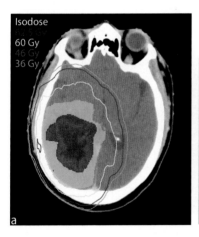
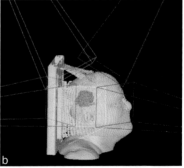

FIGURE 3.1 (a) A 55-year-old man with right parietal glioblastoma (GBM) with spread through the corpus callosum, s/p stereotactic biopsy. GTV based on contrast enhancement in red, and T2/FLAIR changes in green. EBRT: 60 Gy/2 Gy/fx, via 5-field IMRT; 6 MV photons prescribed to the 98% IDL. 60 Gy IDL in yellow. (b) Beam arrangement for this patient. Non-coplanar, 5-field plan. T1 contrast enhancement in red, T2/FLAIR in green. *Continued on next page.*

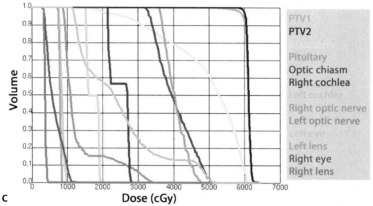

PTV1
PTV2
Brainstem
Pituitary
Optic chiasm
Right cochlea
Left cochlea
Right optic nerve
Left optic nerve
Left eye
Left lens
Right eye
Right lens

c

FIGURE 3.1 (c) DVH for this patient. Note: dose constraints adapted to avoid compromising dose to treatment volume. (d) A 31-year-old woman with a left fronto-parietal low-grade glioma per stereotactic biopsy. The radiographic enhancement is highly suggestive of high-grade astrocytoma. T2 signal change with a 2-cm margin for CTV and 5-mm margin for PTV in green. T1 contrast enhancement with 1-cm margin for CTV and 5-mm margin for PTV in red. T2 signal change PTV treated to 50.4 Gy followed by a 9-Gy boost to the area of contrast enhancement plus 1-cm margin for CTV and 5-mm margin for PTV.

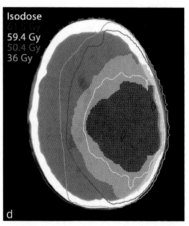

Isodose
61.5 Gy
59.4 Gy
50.4 Gy
36 Gy

d

GLIOMA—LOW GRADE

Indications and Options for Treatment

■ Definitive therapy.
■ Adjuvant therapy in the postoperative setting.

Localization, Immobilization, Simulation for Fractionated RT/FSRT

■ Per general principles.

Volumes, Dose, and Fractionation

■ Volumes (see Figure 3.2)

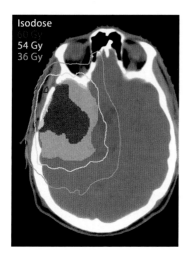

Isodose
60 Gy
54 Gy
36 Gy

FIGURE 3.2 A 22-year-old right-handed man with right temporal low-grade mixed glioma, near-total resection 2.5 years ago, now progression. EBRT alone: 54 Gy/1.8 Gy/fx, via 5-field IMRT, mix 6/10 MV photons prescribed to the 97% IDL. T2 signal change in red, PTV in green = GTV + 2 cm (CTV), then + 0.3 cm (PTV). 54 Gy IDL in yellow.

- GTV: signal change on T2 MRI
- CTV: GTV + 1.5 to 2 cm
- PTV: CTV + 0.5 cm
- Dose and fractionation
  - 54 Gy/1.8 Gy/fx

Special Considerations

- Treat gemistocytic astrocytoma as per anaplastic astrocytoma.

BRAINSTEM GLIOMA

Indications for Treatment

- Radiotherapy is standard treatment for inoperable brainstem glioma.
- Lesions are usually not biopsied.

Localization, Immobilization, Simulation for Fractionated RT/FSRT

- Per general principles.

Volumes, Dose, and Fractionation

- Volumes (see Figure 3.3)
  - GTV: greatest dimension on T1 or T2 MRI.
  - CTV: GTV + 2-cm margin with respect for natural boundaries.
  - PTV: CTV + 0.3 to 0.5 cm margin with respect for natural boundaries.
- Dose and fractionation
  - 54 Gy/1.8 Gy/fx

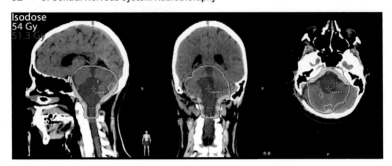

FIGURE 3.3 A 21-year-old woman with brain stem low-grade oligodendroglioma, 1p19q intact, status-post biopsy. GTV in red by all MRI sequences. PTV in blue (GTV + 2 cm margin; + 0.3 cm margin for PTV). EBRT: 54 Gy/1.8 Gy/fx, via 7-field IMRT with 6 MV photons prescribed to 100% IDL.

MENINGIOMA

Indications for Treatment

- Benign: inoperability or subtotal resection.
- Atypical: inoperability, status-post gross total resection, status-post subtotal resection.
- Malignant: inoperability, status-post gross total resection, status-post subtotal resection.

Localization, Immobilization, Simulation for Fractionated RT/FSRT

- Per general principles.

Volumes, Dose, and Fractionation

- Volumes (see Figure 3.4a)
  - GTV: enhancement on T1 MRI
  - CTV: GTV = CTV
  - PTV: CTV + 0.3 to 0.5 cm
- Dose and fractionation (definitive)
  - Benign: 54 Gy/1.8 Gy/fx
    - GTV: enhancement on T1 MRI
    - CTV: GTV = CTV
    - PTV: CTV + 0.3 to 0.5 cm
  - Atypical: 59.4 Gy/1.8 Gy/fx.
    - GTV: enhancement on T1 MRI
    - CTV: GTV + 1 cm with respect for natural barriers
    - PTV: CTV + 0.3 to 0.5 cm
  - Malignant: 59.4 to 60 Gy/1.8 to 2 Gy/fx.

- GTV: enhancement on T1 MRI
- CTV: GTV + 2 cm with respect for natural barriers
- PTV: CTV + 0.3 to 0.5 cm
■ Dose and fractionation (postoperative)
  ■ Benign: 54 Gy/1.8 Gy/fx for subtotal resection
    - GTV: enhancement on T1 MRI
    - CTV: GTV = CTV
    - PTV: CTV + 0.3 to 0.5 cm
  ■ Atypical: 54 Gy/1.8 Gy/fx for gross total resection and 59.4 Gy/1.8 Gy/fx for subtotal resection
    - GTV: enhancement on T1 MRI
    - CTV: GTV + 1 cm with respect for natural barriers

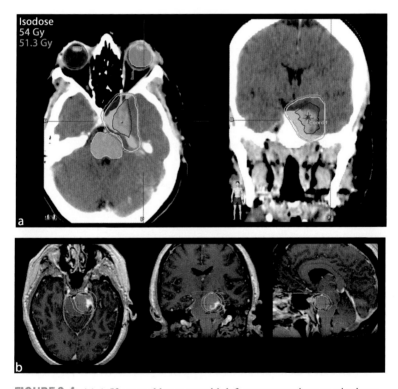

FIGURE 3.4 (a) A 53-year-old woman with left cavernous sinus meningioma. On axial and coronal images, GTV (area of contrast enhancement) in red. EBRT: 54 Gy/1.8 Gy/fx, via 7-field IMRT with 6 MV photons prescribed to the 100% IDL. (b) A 40-year-old woman with left tentorial meningioma with brainstem compression, status-post subtotal resection treated with gamma knife (GK) SRS, 12 Gy prescribed to the 50% IDL, seen in yellow.

- PTV: CTV + 0.3 to 0.5 cm
- Malignant: 59.4 to 60 Gy /1.8 to 2 Gy/fx for both gross and subtotal resections
  - GTV: enhancement on T1 MRI
  - CTV: GTV + 2 cm with respect for natural barriers
  - PTV: CTV + 0.3 to 0.5 cm
- SRS (see Figure 3.4b) may be used if:
  - The lesion is more than 0.3 to 0.5 cm away from the optic chiasm.
  - The dose is 13 to 14 Gy (higher doses may be considered for atypical and malignant meningiomas).
  - Optic chiasm dose is limited to 8 to 9 Gy with consideration that some institutions accept higher doses to the optic chiasm.

Special Considerations

- Inclusion of dural tail is controversial, particularly with regard to SRS.
- Care must be taken for parasagittal lesions as malignant edema may occur with treatment of parasagittal meningiomas.

PITUITARY ADENOMA

Indications for Treatment

- Unresectable or subtotally resected lesions.
- SRS is the preferred treatment modality.

Localization, Immobilization, Simulation for Fractionated RT/FSRT

- Per general principles.

Volumes, Dose, and Fractionation

Fractionated radiotherapy
- Volumes (see Figure 3.5)
  - GTV: gadolinium enhancement on T1 MRI with contrast
  - CTV: GTV = CTV
  - PTV: CTV + 0.5 cm
- Dose and fractionation
  - 45 Gy/1.8 Gy/fx for nonfunctional pituitary adenoma and 50.4 Gy/1.8 Gy/fx for secretory adenomas.
- SRS
  - Preferred treatment modality.
  - Feasible if lesion is more than 0.3 to 0.5 cm away from the optic chiasm.
  - Dose
    - 15 to 16 Gy for nonfunctional adenomas
    - 18 to 25 Gy for secretory adenomas

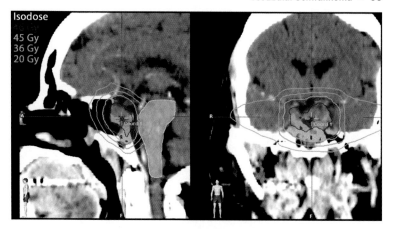

FIGURE 3.5 A 61-year-old woman with nonsecreting pituitary macroadenoma, status-post transsphenoidal resection 14 years prior to recurrence. Recurrence treated with subtotal transsphenoidal reresection followed by 45 Gy/1.8 Gy/fx IMRT, via an 8-field technique with 6 MV photons prescribed to the 100% IDL.

VESTIBULAR SCHWANNOMA

Indications for Radiotherapy Treatment

- To maintain hearing.
- Radiographic progression.

Localization, Immobilization, Simulation for Fractionated RT/FSRT

- Per general principles.

Volumes, Dose, and Fractionation

- Volumes (see Figure 3.4)
  - GTV: T1-weighted enhancing tumor
  - CTV: GTV = CTV
  - PTV: CTV + 0.5 cm for fractionated EBRT, PTV = CTV for SRS
  - Contour applicable regions of interest as seen in Table 3.1
- Dose (see Figure 3.6)
  - 45 to 54 Gy/1.8 Gy/fx
  - SRS dose 13 Gy to 50% IDL with gamma knife SRS (Figure 3.6) and 80% IDL with linear accelerator (LINAC) SRS
- Fractionation

- Fractionated EBRT or FSRT for tumors ≥3.5 cm or normal/minimal hearing loss and SRS for lesions smaller than 3.5 cm.

Special Considerations

- Patients with neurofibromatosis-2 are often affected by bilateral vestibular schwannomas (synchronously or metachronously), increasing the risk for bilateral deafness.
- Consider fractionated EBRT, as it may allow greater hearing preservation than SRS.

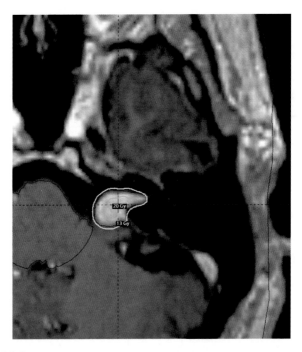

FIGURE 3.6 Left vestibular schwannoma with classic "ice cream cone" shape. Treated with GK SRS, 13 Gy to the 50% IDL. Yellow: 50% IDL; green: 100% IDL.

ARTERIOVENOUS MALFORMATION

Indications and Options for Treatment

- Reduce the risk of hemorrhage and neurologic deficits/symptoms.
- Spetzler-Martin I and II—surgical intervention preferred for faster decline of risk of hemorrhage.
- Spetzler-Martin grade III—surgical intervention versus SRS with consideration for factors included in Spetzler-Martin grading system (size, eloquence, and venous drainage) as they apply to an individual case.
- Spetzler-Martin grade IV/V—staged radiosurgery with multiple isocenters may be feasible for select large lesions (1).

Localization, Immobilization, Simulation

- Per general principles.

Volumes, Dose, and Fractionation

- Volume
  - As delineated on high-volume MRI and angiogram.
- Dose
  - 14 to 27 Gy

Special Considerations

- Aneurysms on feeding arteries of arteriovenous malformations must be addressed prior to interventions on the arteriovenous malformation nidus to avoid increased arterial pressure at the site of aneurysm following arteriovenous malformation nidus ablation.

SPINAL CORD TUMORS

Indications and Options for Treatment

- Adjuvant or definitive treatment.
- In the setting of inoperability or low-grade gliomas, particularly in young children, it is reasonable to attempt to delay radiotherapy as long as is feasible.

Localization, Immobilization, Simulation for Fractionated RT/FSRT

- Positioning: supine with arms at the side.
- Localization: coregister planning CT with preoperative T1 and T2 MRI to delineate GTV.
- Immobilization: vacuum bag device.

TABLE 3.2 Approach to Spinal Cord Tumors

Histology	Surgery	Adjuvant Treatment
Low-grade astrocytoma (WHO I-II)	Attempt GTR (mostly obtained with pilocytic astro)	GTR: none STR/Biopsy (Bx): focal EBRT to 50.4-54 Gy
High-grade astrocytoma (WHO III-IV)	Bx or STR (difficult to resect because of infiltrative nature)	Focal RT to 50.4 Gy (CTV) with boost to 54-59.4 (GTV), consider chemotherapy
Meningioma	Attempt GTR	GTR: none STR/Bx: observation (low grade [LG]) vs focal EBRT to 54 Gy
Schwannoma/ neurofibroma	Attempt GTR (frequently need to sacrifice nerve)	GTR: none STR/Bx: 50.4-54 Gy /1.8 Gy/ fx. Consider SRS for skull base (Florida).
Hemangioma	GTR (for cord compression)	GTR: none None (or failed embolization, ethanol injection, vertebro-plasty), symptomatic: focal EBRT to 40 Gy at 2 Gy/fx.
Spinal canal (ie, neurofibrosarcoma/ malignant peripheral nerve shealth tumor (MPNST)	Attempt GTR (infrequently obtained)	Charged particles to 60-70 Gy +/- chemotherapy. Consider IMRT.
Vertebral body (ie, chondrosarcoma, chordoma, osteogenic sarcoma)	Attempt GTR (infrequently obtained)	Charged particles to 70-78 Gy postoperation +/- chemotherapy. Consider IMRT Consider protons.

- Simulation: high-resolution CT scan with or without IV contrast.
  - For lesions located in the superior spine, the cerebellum should be included through at least two vertebrae inferior to the lesion.
  - For lesions located in the inferior spine, the entire sacrum should be included through at least two vertebrae superior to the lesion.
- Planning
  - For spinal cord tumors, contour normal structures in the treatment field and follow dose constraints as per tolerance (see appropriate chapter).

Volumes, Dose, and Fractionation

- Low-grade gliomas:
    - GTV: preoperative signal change on T2 MRI.
    - CTV: GTV + 0.5 to 1 cm cephalad/caudad with radial margins to include nerve roots.
    - PTV: CTV + 0.3 to 0.5 cm.
- High-grade gliomas (Table 3.2):
    - GTV: preoperative enhancing volume on T1 gadolinium contrasted MRI.
    - CTV: GTV + 1.5 cm cephalad/caudad with radial margins to include nerve roots.
    - PTV: CTV + 0.3 to 0.5 cm.
- Include cyst or syrinx volumes in GTV if involved by tumor.
- CSI for grossly disseminated disease.

REFERENCE

1. Spetzler RF, Martin NA. A proposed grading system for arteriovenous malformations. *J Neurosurg.* 1986;65:476–483.

4 Head and Neck Radiotherapy

**Shlomo A. Koyfman, John F. Greskovich, and
Jerrold P. Saxton**

GENERAL PRINCIPLES

- Radical radiotherapy is indicated either in the primary management of head and neck (H&N) cancer (with concurrent chemotherapy for locally advanced disease) or in the postoperative setting (+/− concurrent chemotherapy) if there are high-risk features (eg, T3/4, N2/3, close/+ margins, + extracapsular extension (ECE), recurrent disease).

Localization, Immobilization, and Simulation

- Historically, 2D simulation and field delineation based on anatomic landmarks were very reproducible and effective.
- CT–based volumetric treatment planning is now preferred for definition of GTV, CTV, and PTV.
- Patient position is generally supine with arms at the sides, shoulders relaxed downward, and neck neutral or extended.
- Immobilization involves 3-point thermoplastic head mask; 5-point head and shoulder mask preferred for IMRT. Tongue depressor (aka intraoral stent) helps stabilize tongue and separate palate from the tongue.
- Consider coaching patients to not swallow while the beam is on to avoid tongue/larynx motion, especially for 3D boost fields or IMRT.
- Contiguous spiral CT slices are acquired with 3-mm slice acquisition from the top of the brain through the upper mediastinum.
- Consider IV contrast to delineate major blood vessels.
- The role of PET in delineating the GTV is controversial.
  - Some studies suggest that PET may decrease the primary GTV by 10% to 50% and increase the nodal GTV by identifying lymph nodes negative by CT criteria (1).

Target Volumes and Organs of Interest Definition

- Reference should be made to the 1993 ICRU report no. 62 for complete description of various target volume definitions (GTV, CTV, and PTV).
- GTV: gross tumor as defined by clinical examination and radiographic studies at the primary and LN (CT criteria: >1 cm in short axis or central necrosis). The use of PET in target delineation is controversial.
- CTV: consider the extent of local tumor extension and site-specific patterns of spread.
- PTV: accounts for daily setup error and organ motion. Be mindful of anatomic changes during the course of treatment (eg, tumor shrinkage and weight loss).
- Normal anatomy to be routinely identified
  - Spinal cord (top C1 through T4/5)
  - Glottic larynx
  - Brachial plexus (especially in presence of low lying neck disease)
  - Mandible, temporo-mandibular joint (TMJ)
- Normal anatomy to be identified when treating the base of the skull
  - Brainstem
  - Optic nerves/chiasm
  - Eyes

- Lenses
- Pituitary gland
- Middle/inner ears (or cochlea)
- Additional normal anatomy to be identified when using IMRT
  - Parotid glands
  - Oral cavity
  - Lips
  - Skin (in region of target volumes)
  - Cervical esophagus
  - All unidentified tissue
- Optional normal anatomy that may be identified
  - Submandibular glands
  - Uninvolved pharyngeal constrictor muscles (aka OAR pharynx)

Treatment Planning—Definitive Radiotherapy

External Beam Therapy

- 3-Field approach: in general, opposed laterals are matched to an anterior supraclavicular field to cover primary site and cervical/supraclavicular (SCV) LN at risk.

  Standard lateral field borders (Figure 4.1a)
  - Superior: mastoid tip to cover level II, or the base of the skull, to cover retropharyngeal nodes when indicated.

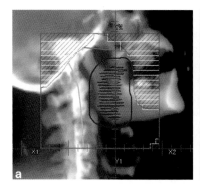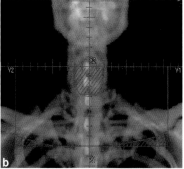

FIGURE 4.1 A 62-year-old man with cT3N2a SCC of the R base of the tongue for definitive chemoradiation. (a) DRR of the lateral field. Purple denotes the original field, green denotes the off-cord field, blue denotes cone down no. 1, and red denotes final cone down. (b) DRR of the anteroposterior low-neck field. Larynx block is in place throughout treatment.

- Inferior: above the arytenoids when the larynx is not involved; if the larynx cannot be spared, place the inferior border below the cricoid (or as low as shoulders permit).
- Anterior: 2 to 3 cm anterior to the tumor, or enough to cover Ib nodes when indicated (anterior border of ramus of mandible).
  - Spare small strip of skin anteriorly (below mandibular area) unless tumor extends to subcutaneous tissue or there are large submandibular/jugular LN.
- Posterior: behind spinous process of C2 when covering level V or at the posterior edge of the vertebral body (off cord) when level V is not included in the field.
  - Move posterior border "off cord" to mid-vertebral body at 42 to 44 Gy.
  - Supplement blocked portion of off-cord field with posterior en face electrons.

Posterior en face electron field (aka "post strips")
- Superior, posterior, inferior: same as initial lateral fields (or may add 5-10 mm to account for "bowing in" of high isodose lines with electrons)
- Anterior
  - abutting posterior border of off-cord field ("hot match")—confirm light fields
  - or alternatively may leave 2- to 3-mm gap to avoid hotspot if lymphatics are adequately covered at depth as per the plan

Standard anteroposterior field borders (Figure 4.1b)
- Superior: matched to the inferior border of lateral fields
- Inferior: 1 cm below the clavicles
- Lateral: cover medial two thirds of the clavicle
- Blocks: include a larynx block throughout treatment when not at risk. Include full midline (spinal cord) block if treating anteroposterior (AP) field above 50 Gy. When the larynx block is contraindicated, consider 0.5- to 1-cm cord block on the lateral field to avoid excessive spinal cord dose from field overlap. If a single isocentric technique used, this block may be omitted.

Boost field borders
- Primary site dependent
- Treat tumor + 1- to 2-cm margin with reduced opposed lateral or oblique fields.
- Enlarged LN can be treated with an appositional electron beam field or opposed oblique (off cord) fields if neck dissection is not planned.

Optional cone down no. 1 borders (for intermediate risk areas)
- Consider for infiltrative lesions with ill-defined borders to ensure adequate coverage of subclinical disease.

- Cover primary tumor with expanded margins (1.5-2 cm) prior to final cone down.
- IMRT
  - Primary reference: because IMRT is a relatively novel treatment modality for H&N malignancies, treatment is guided by practice consensus as reflected in many of the RTOG protocols, which will be liberally cited.
  - Nomenclature: there are a variety of ways to refer to the finalized volumes used in IMRT planning.
    - The CTV/PTV expansion of the GTV may be referred to as:
      - CTV1/PTV1
      - CTV-high dose (CTV_{HD})/PTV-high dose (PTV_{HD})
      - High-risk CTV/high-risk PTV
      - CTV_{dose}/ PTV_{dose}, eg, CTV_{70}/PTV_{70}
    - The CTV/PTV, which includes elective/low-risk nodes, can be referred to as:
      - CTV2/PTV2
      - CTV-elective dose (CTV-ED)/PTV-elective dose (PTV-ED)
      - Low-risk CTV/low-risk PTV
      - CTV_{dose}/ PTV_{dose}, eg, $CTV_{59.4}$/$PTV_{59.4}$
    - The CTV/PTV expansion of the intermediate risk used by some radiation oncologists can be referred to as:
      - CTV_{INT} /PTV_{INT}
      - CTV_{dose}/ PTV_{dose}, eg, CTV_{63}/PTV_{63}
  - Technique: use the same principles as outlined above to identify areas at risk and clarify the dose needed based on nature of risk (involved vs elective) (Figure 4.2a and b)
    - Definition of the GTV: as above.
    - Definition of the CTV_{HD}: GTV + 5 to 10 mm. Can be reduced to 1 mm when abutting critical normal tissues (eg, tumor invading clivus and abutting brainstem).
    - Definition of CTV_{ED}: all clinically negative, elective nodal areas felt to be at risk of microscopic tumor involvement plus an additional 5- to 10-mm margin around CTV_{HD}. See RTOG nodal atlas for aid in delineating nodal stations (note: atlas developed for node-negative patients; http://208.251.169.72/atlases/hnatlas/main.html).
    - Definition of the CTV_{INT}: if GTV margin is ill-defined (infiltrative tumor), one may consider an intermediate dose to a 1-cm margin of tissue surrounding selective areas of CTV_{HD}.
    - Definition of the PTV: CTV + 5 mm (ie, PTV_{HD}, CTV_{HD} + 5 mm; PTV_{ED}, CTV_{ED} + 5 mm). May be reduced to 3 mm with adequate image-guided radiation therapy.

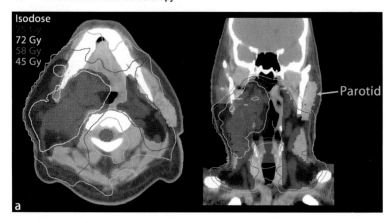

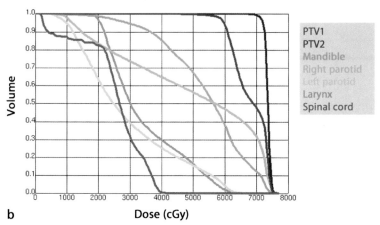

FIGURE 4.2 A 53-year-old man with a cT2N3M0 SCC of the R tonsil for definitive chemoradiation. (a) Axial and coronal images displaying isodose distributions. Shaded red is PTVHD, shaded blue is PTVED. (b) DVH of treatment plan.

Brachytherapy

- Historically used for oral cavity lesions, base of tongue (BOT) or nasopharyngeal boost, and recurrent disease.
  - Target is identified (marked before external beam in case of regression), and implant is designed.
  - Single-plane implant for smaller lesions less than 5 to 10 mm in width. Double-plane implant for 10- to 20-mm lesions. Volumetric implant for anything bigger or irregularly shaped.
  - Needle spacing is typically 10 mm.

Treatment Planning—Postoperative Radiotherapy

- Both for 3D planning and IMRT, the guiding principles and field design are similar to the definitive setting, with the exception of the lack of a GTV.
- In general, the CTV encompasses the primary tumor bed (based on preoperative imaging, preoperative physical examination and endoscopy, and operative and pathologic findings), any pathologically involved nodal

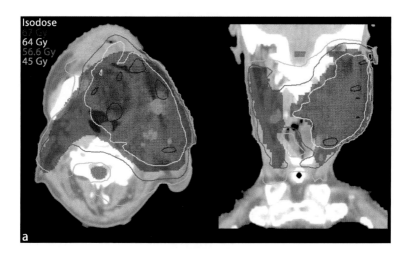

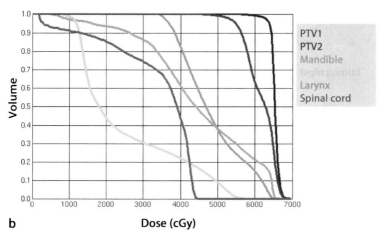

FIGURE 4.3 A 66-year-old man with pT4N2bM0 SCC of the L base of tongue s/p tracheotomy, resection, and free flap reconstruction treated with postoperative chemoradiation. (a) Axial and coronal images displaying isodose distribution. Shaded red is PTV$_{HD}$, shaded blue is PTV$_{ED}$. (b) DVH of treatment plan.

stations, and elective nodal stations, when clinically indicated (Figure 4.3a and b). Consider treating elective areas to lower dose (CTV_{ED}), and boosting areas at very high risk (eg. + margins).

Dose/Fractionation

Definitive (Chemo)radiotherapy setting

- Once-daily fractionation (doses are assuming 2 Gy/fx; 1.8 Gy/fx can also be used, if preferred):
  - 50 to 54 Gy to elective nodal areas.
  - Off-cord field at 42 Gy using photon fields anterior to cord and en face electrons to posterior cervical nodal chain to a dose of 50 to 54 Gy.
  - Consider optional cone down no. 1 to 64 Gy for tumors with ill-defined margins.
  - Boost GTV to 70 to 74 Gy.
- Twice-daily fractionation
  - 55.2 Gy/1.2 Gy/fx to elective nodal areas.
  - Off-cord field at 43.2 Gy using photon fields anterior to cord and en face electrons to posterior cervical nodal chain to dose of 55.2 Gy.
  - Consider optional cone down no. 1 to 64.8 Gy/1.2 Gy/fx for tumors with ill-defined margins.
  - Boost GTV to 74.4 to 76.8 Gy/1.2 Gy/fx.
  - Treat with at least a 6-hour interfraction interval.
- Concomitant boost technique (per RTOG 0522)
  - 54 Gy/1.8 Gy/fx to elective nodal areas.
  - Off-cord field at 41.4 Gy using photon fields anterior to cord and en face electrons to posterior cervical nodal chain.
  - At least 50.4 Gy to 3-cm depth of the posterior neck (when clinically negative) delivered with posterior en face electrons.
  - At 32.4 Gy, begin concomitant boost to GTV and involved nodes with 1.5 Gy/fx as a second daily fraction for the final 12 treatment days (18 Gy); total dose is 72 Gy.
  - Consider optional cone down no. 1 by delivering 1.5 Gy in 6 fx to dose of 63 Gy prior to final cone down.
  - Treat with at least a 6-hour interfraction interval.
- IMRT technique (Table 4.1)
- For all approaches: low anterior field is treated with monoisocentrically matched AP or AP/posteroanterior fields to 50 to 50.4 Gy/1.8 to 2 Gy/fx delivered to a 3-cm depth when clinically uninvolved. If gross disease exists in low neck, can deliver 69 to 72 Gy if able to limit brachial plexus to 60 Gy or less. Otherwise, treat to 60 Gy with planned neck dissection, regardless of response. (See below for discussion of matching techniques under "IMRT: Field Matching Techniques" section).

TABLE 4.1 IMRT Technique

Per RTOG 0522 (6 Fractions Weekly)	Per RTOG 0615 (5 Fractions Weekly)
Sites: oropharynx, hypopharynx, larynx	Site: nasopharynx
PTV_{HD} treated to 70 Gy/2 Gy/fx	PTV_{70} treated to 70 Gy/2.12 Gy/fx
PTV_{ED} treated to 56 Gy/1.6 Gy/fx	$PTV_{59.4}$ treated to 59.4 Gy/1.8 Gy/fx
PTV_{INT} (optional), 59.5–63 Gy/ 1.7–1.8 Gy/fx	PTV_{63} (optional), 63 Gy/1.9 Gy/fx

- When using IMRT, one can alternatively treat primary, upper, and lower neck using a single IMRT plan with appropriate laryngeal constraints (mean dose, <45 Gy if possible).

Postoperative setting
- 60 Gy to tumor bed and involved nodes. Consider 56 Gy to elective nodes.
- Consider boosting high-risk areas (known ECE and/or microscopically positive margins) to 66 Gy.

Critical Structures* (in order of descending planning importance) (Table 4.2)

Technical Factors
- 3D CRT
    - Use 6 MV photons for laterals and SCV fields. Prescribe SCV field to a depth of 3 cm if no GTV in field.
    - Can consider higher energy photons from uninvolved side for boost in order to spare superficial tissue, including the mandible. Alternatively, consider weighting fields (3:2) toward the affected side for boost.
    - For posterior en face electron field, use 9 to 12 MeV electrons; use higher energy electrons for muscular patients or bulky, involved nodes.
    - Doses are to be calculated *with* heterogeneity corrections.
- IMRT
    - Planning goals
        - At least 95% of the PTV receives the prescription dose (V100 ≥ 95%).
        - At least 99% of the PTV should receive greater than 93% of the pre-scribed dose (V93 ≥ 99%).
        - No more than 20% of PTV will receive 110% or greater of the pre-scription dose (V110 ≤ 20%).

TABLE 4.2   Critical Structures* (In Order of Descending Planning Importance)

Spinal cord	No more than 0.03 cc can receive =48 Gy
Brainstem	54 Gy
Optic chiasm/nerves	50 Gy
Brachial plexus	=60 Gy preferred, 66 Gy maximum
Glottic larynx	Mean dose <45 Gy
Mandible, tempero-mandibular joint	=70 Gy preferred; no more than 1 cc, >75 Gy
Unspecified tissue (outside targets)	No more than 5% can receive >prescription dose; no more than 1% or 1 cc of unspecified tissue can receive =110% of the prescription dose.
Parotid gland	Mean dose to at least 1 gland =26 Gy OR at least 20 cc of the combined volume of both parotid glands to <20 Gy OR at least 50% of 1 gland to <30 Gy
Oral cavity minus PTV	Mean dose <40 Gy
Lips	Mean dose <20; maximum dose <30 (<50 for oral cavity lesions)
Cochlea	No more than 5% >55 Gy
Eyes	Maximum dose <50 Gy
Lens	Maximum dose <25 Gy
Esophagus/postcricoid pharynx/OAR pharynx	Mean dose <45 Gy

*These constraints are all per RTOG protocols.

- No more than 5% of PTV will receive 115% or greater of the prescription dose (V115 ≤ 5%).
  - Field matching considerations: for lesions above the larynx, can match IMRT field to conventional low anterior neck field or can use a single IMRT plan.
    - Advantages to single IMRT field is the lack of hot/cold spots at the junction (can be up to 20%), but at the expense of less laryngeal shielding.
    - Advantages to matched fields is better laryngeal shielding and may improve IMRT plan to primary tumor region, but at the expense of junction changes and significant risk of hot/cold spots at match line.
    - The primary technique to accomplish an IMRT/AP field match is to use a *half-beam block/monoisocentric technique*. Close inferior jaw to the central axis for IMRT field and vice versa for the AP field. Feath-

ering the junction superior/inferior 3 mm, twice during treatment, is recommended to reduce hot/cold spots at the junction.

- Alternative techniques to avoid the need to feather the junction include the following:
  - Dynamic field matching technique: involves continuously moving the superior border of the AP field from 1.5 cm below the central axis (ie, match line) to 1.5 cm above the central axis, creating in effect a 3-cm match line (2). No field junctions are necessary.
  - "Gradient matching" technique: involves modifying the superior border of the AP field so that the total dose per fraction (eg, 2 Gy) is delivered in 3 separate segments, with only about one third of the dose delivered at the superior most aspect of the original field. This creates a broad dose gradient along the match line (no field junctions necessary). One must be careful to extend the IMRT target volume 1 to 2 cm into the AP field to ensure that the inverse planning system accounts for this deliberate "underdosing" and ensures adequate coverage (3).
- Replanning
  - Patient/tumor geometry frequently changes during the course of treatment because of tumor and normal tissue shrinkage and/or weight loss of the patient. As such, some advocate for replanning during the course of therapy, particularly for IMRT planning, where dosimetric goals may be significantly compromised with even small anatomic changes given the steep dose gradients.
  - Whereas some have found significant overdosing of critical structures without replanning (4), others have found the impact of replanning to be limited to parotid sparing only (5).
  - Both the need to replan and the ideal frequency of replanning remain an area of controversy and active investigation.

OROPHARYNX CANCER

Site-Specific Indications

- Radiotherapy (+/- chemotherapy) is indicated for an organ preservation treatment approach.

Target Volumes

- GTV/PTV: as per general principles.
- CTV: draining lymphatics include levels II to IV and retropharyngeal/parapharyngeal nodes for all cases. Include level Ib if BOT, tonsil, or upper jugular nodes are involved. Include level V for any N+ or tonsil/BOT primary.

Special Considerations

- For well-lateralized T1-2/N0-1 tonsil tumors, can consider unilateral irradiation, including primary tumor + ipsilateral levels II to IV only. Can use mixed electron-photon beam (4:1) with open neck technique (tumors <5 cm deep), wedged pair in supine position (tumors >5 cm deep), or IMRT (Figure 4.4).

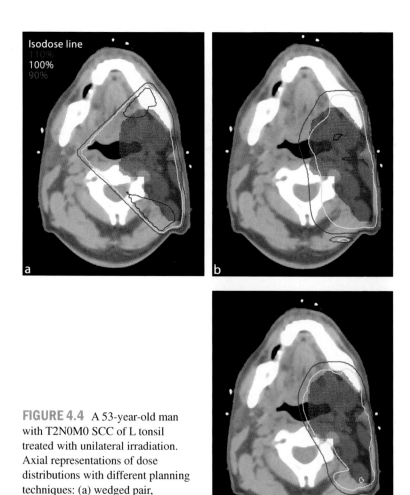

FIGURE 4.4 A 53-year-old man with T2N0M0 SCC of L tonsil treated with unilateral irradiation. Axial representations of dose distributions with different planning techniques: (a) wedged pair, (b) mixed photon-electron (1:4), (c) IMRT. Shaded red is PTV$_{HD}$, shaded blue is PTV$_{ED}$.

- For pharyngeal wall tumor, inferior border is extended more than 3 cm beyond the pharyngeal wall mass to include the entire pharynx in initial fields; the posterior border for the tumor boost/cone down is placed immediately anterior to the spinal cord. Daily verification images are required to verify setup.
- For any bulky posterior cervical neck disease, can rotate the gantry for laterals to ensure adequate coverage while still protecting spinal cord.

LARYNX CANCER

Site-Specific Indications

- Radiotherapy alone is the standard treatment for early glottic cancer. Concurrent chemoradiotherapy is indicated for laryngeal preservation in locally advanced disease. For patients with extensive bone/cartilage involvement, total laryngectomy + postoperative (chemo)radiotherapy is preferred.

Target Volumes

- Early-stage glottic cancer (T1/2, N0)
  - For early-stage glottic tumor (T1/2, N0), no elective nodal irradiation is required. Field is generally 5 × 5 or 6 × 6 cm with opposed laterals (Figure 4.5a and b). Consider unilateral field for disease involving 1 cord only (Figure 4.5c).
  - Borders are as follows:
    - Superior: top of thyroid cartilage for T1, additional 1 cm higher for T2.
    - Anterior: flash anteriorly.
    - Posterior: anterior margin of vertebral bodies. Some advocate a cone down where this border is moved anteriorly by 0.5 to 1 cm to spare some of the arytenoids and avoid late laryngeal edema. This can be done only in the absence of gross disease in the posterior half of the vocal cords (Figure 4.5d).
    - Inferior: lower edge of cricoid cartilage for T1, as low as possible without treating through the shoulders for T2.
  - Intensity-modulated radiation therapy is not recommended in this setting.
  - Consider nodal irradiation for extensive supraglottic/subglottic extension as risk of occult nodal metastases is higher.
- All other larynx cancer
  - GTV/PTV: as per general principles.
  - CTV: draining lymphatics include levels II to IV. Include level V for any N+ or extension to the BOT. Include retropharyngeal nodes if extension to pharyngeal wall (possibly glossopharyngeal sulcus) or BOT.

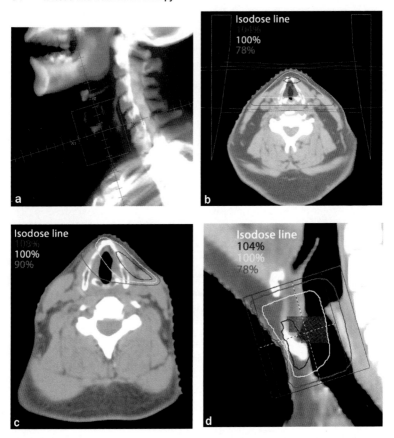

FIGURE 4.5 A 53-year-old man with T1N0 SCC of the L true vocal cord for definitive radiation. (a) DRR of lateral field. (b) Axial representations of dose distribution with opposed laterals with wedges. (c) Axial representation of dose distribution with unilateral field only. (d) Sagittal demonstration of lateral field with optional cone down to reduce dose to arytenoids.

Special Considerations

- For early-stage glottic cancer (T1, N0), hypofractionation has been shown to improve local control compared with standard fractionation. Recommended dose is 63 Gy/2.25 Gy/fx or 66 Gy/2.2 Gy/fx.
- For T2, N0 glottic cancer, especially lesions with impaired vocal cord mobility (T2b disease), consider treating to 65.25 Gy/2.25 Gy/fx or to 74.4 Gy/1.2 Gy/fx twice daily, or accelerated concomitant boost technique, or

treating with 6 fx weekly. Some advocate the addition of radiosensitizing chemotherapy in this setting.

■ After total laryngectomy, include tracheal stoma if subglottic extension, emergency tracheostomy through tumor, tumor invasion into soft tissue of neck (including ECE), + tracheal margin, or surgical scar crosses the stoma.

HYPOPHARYNX CANCER

Site-Specific Indications

■ Concurrent chemoradiotherapy is indicated for organ preservation in advanced disease. For patients with extensive bone/cartilage involvement, total laryngopharyngectomy + postoperative (chemo)radiotherapy is preferred.

Target Volumes

■ GTV/PTV: as per general principles.
■ CTV
  ■ CTV_{HD} = GTV + 5 mm
  ■ CTV_{ED} includes bilateral levels Ib to V, and retropharyngeal/parapharyngeal nodes for all cases.

Special Considerations

■ Care must be taken not to underestimate the inferior extent of the disease (toward the apex) because it is very difficult to appreciate on endoscopic exam or on imaging. If matching laterals/IMRT to AP field, match below the cricoids, or as low as necessary, to achieve margin on disease (do not match over tumor). Including superior esophagus may be necessary.

NASOPHARYNX CANCER

Site-Specific Indications

■ Definitive chemoradiotherapy is standard for nasopharyngeal cancer of all stages.

Target Volumes

■ GTV/PTV: as per general principles. MRI fusion is recommended to help delineate intracranial organs at risk and areas of tumor infiltration and helps visualize nerves that need to be included.

- CTV
  - CTV_{HD} = GTV + 5 mm
  - CTV_{ED} (per RTOG 0615) = the entire nasopharynx, anterior one half to two thirds of the clivus (entire clivus, if involved), skull base (foramen ovale and rotundum bilaterally must be included for all cases), pterygoid fossae, parapharyngeal space, inferior sphenoid sinus (in T3-T4 disease, the entire sphenoid sinus), and posterior fourth to third of the nasal cavity and maxillary sinuses (to ensure pterygopalatine fossae coverage). The cavernous sinus should be included in high-risk patients (T3, T4, bulky disease involving the roof of the nasopharynx). Draining lymphatics include bilateral levels Ib to V and retropharyngeal/parapharyngeal nodes for all cases.

Special Considerations

- Level Ib nodes may be spared in node-negative patients, or node + only in retropharyngeal or level IV nodes.
- If hard palate, nasal cavity, or maxillary antrum is involved, bilateral IB nodes must be covered.
- CTV_{HD} margin can be reduced to 1 mm for tumors in close proximity to critical structures (eg, tumor invading clivus and abutting, but not involving, brainstem). However, CTV_{HD} margin should not be reduced if disease is frankly invading the critical structure.

MAJOR SALIVARY GLAND CANCER

Site-Specific Indications

- Radiotherapy is generally indicated in the postoperative setting and for locally advanced disease (T3/4, N+) or T1/2, N0 with high-risk features (high grade, + margin, peri-neural invasion (PNI), lymphovascular space invasion (LVSI), adenoid cystic histology) or recurrent disease.
- In cases where surgery is not feasible, neutron therapy has shown some advantage.

Target Volumes (Postoperative)

- CTV (parotid)
  - For low-grade, N0 tumors: parotid bed only.
  - For high-grade, N0 tumors (non-adenoid cystic histology): consider electively treating levels Ib, II, III.
  - For N+ tumors: parotid bed + ipsilateral levels I to V.

- For all cases with extensive facial nerve invasion, or adenoid cystic histology, cover facial nerve pathway up to the base of the skull. Focal perineural invasion is not an indication.
- CTV (submandibular)
  - Aside from small, low-grade tumors with N0 neck, cover ipsilateral levels I to IV electively, even in N0 neck. Cover level V if N+. If named nerve is extensively involved (eg, lingual, hypoglossal), cover up to base of skull.
- PTV: as per general principles.

Special Considerations

- Set up patient with "open-neck" technique to expose ipsilateral neck; consider bolus to ensure adequate superficial coverage over surgical bed.
- Intensity-modulated radiation therapy planning is favored for improved homogeneity and reduced dose to contralateral critical structures. Other planning techniques include a wedge pair or mixed photon/electron fields (Figure 4.4).

ORAL CAVITY CANCER
Site-Specific Indications

- Radiotherapy for oral cavity cancers is indicated for use in the postoperative setting for T3/4, pN2/3, close/positive margins, PNI, and +ECE.

Target Volumes (Postoperative)

- CTV: postoperative bed + draining lymphatics include ipsilateral levels Ia/b, II, and III when electively treating. If high-risk disease, or N+, treat ipsilateral levels I to V. Consider contralateral neck irradiation if primary lesion approaches midline (eg, floor of mouth and central mobile tongue).
- PTV: as per general principles.

Special Considerations

- When treating lip (eg, with electrons) or buccal mucosa lesion, consider inserting a lead block (with wax on either side to prevent backscatter) to shield gingiva/teeth/tongue.
- For large (T3) or high-grade T2 upper lip lesions, treat facial lymphatics electively with a moustache field (see image in subsection on nasal cavity).
- For medically inoperable patients, consider a combination of external beam RT (40-50 Gy) + brachytherapy or intraoral cone boost (20-25 Gy).

CANCER OF UNKNOWN PRIMARY

Site-Specific Indications

- Radiotherapy is used for carcinoma of unknown primaries of the H&N region, after neck dissection as primary treatment.

Target Volumes

- CTV: in general, include pharyngeal axis (include base of skull and post one third of the nasal cavity to ensure margin on the nasopharynx) and bilateral levels Ib to V as well as retropharyngeal nodes, with the following exceptions:
  - Squamous cell carcinoma (SCC) found in unilateral level Ib node only: treat bilateral levels I to V.
  - SCC found in 1 parotid LN may be related to primary skin cancer of the scalp: treat ipsilateral levels II to V, parotid, and preauricular nodes. Take skin cancer history and examine scalp for primary lesion.
  - For adenocarcinoma histology metastatic to parotid, parotidectomy is required and helps guide field design.
- PTV: as per general principles.

Special Considerations

- For patients with a single node, without ECE, observation after a neck dissection is recommended.
- Isolated supraclavicular metastases are almost always from a primary below the clavicles, and comprehensive pharyngeal axis irradiation is usually not offered.
- For adenocarcinoma histology, parotidectomy is required and helps guide field design.
- If matching fields via monoisocentric technique, place isocenter as low as possible above the shoulders.

MAXILLARY SINUS CANCER

Site-Specific Indications

- Radiotherapy is indicated in the postoperative setting for all but small, low-grade tumors that have been completely resected with adequate margins.

Target Volumes

- CTV (postoperative)

- MRI fusion is recommended to help delineate intracranial organs at risk and areas of tumor infiltration and helps visualize nerves that need to be included.
- Carefully review operative report for extent of disease spread, paying attention to invasion of orbital wall, cribriform plate, and cranial nerve foramina.
- CTV includes the tumor bed + 1cm margin.
- Consider a boost to high-risk areas (+ margin, PNI) in this volume.

■ PTV: as per general principles. Image-guided radiation therapy is preferred to limit margins and help reduce dose to critical structures (ie, optic nerves).

Special Considerations

- Fill all air cavities or surgical defects with obturator or water-filled balloon to improve dose homogeneity.
- Intensity-modulated radiation therapy planning is preferred given high doses in proximity to critical structures (eg, optic apparatus) (Figure 4.6a and b).
- 3D CRT is delivered (for suprastructure lesions) via a 3-field approach consisting of an AP and opposed laterals (often with 5° post tilt and 60° wedges). Fields are weighted 1.0:0.15:0.15 or 1.0:0.07:0.07. Can consider weighting fields 1:0.5:0.25 where the ipsilateral lateral beam is weighted less heavily (0.25) than the contralateral (0.5). Sequential cone downs may be necessary to avoid high dose to critical structures (frontal lobe if frontal sinus involved; optic apparatus).
- If orbit is uninvolved, treat up to the medial limbus of the eye (exclude lens and retina). If involved, treat the entire eye while trying to shield the lacrimal gland if uninvolved by disease.
- Elective nodal irradiation is controversial in this setting. For N+ disease, treat bilateral IB-V if the patient can tolerate treatment.

NASAL CAVITY/VESTIBULE CANCER

Site-Specific Indications

- Radiotherapy is indicated for smaller lesions (may be cosmetically superior to surgery) or postoperatively for locally advanced lesions.

Target Volumes

- GTV/PTV (definitive): per general principles.
- CTV (nasal vestibule)

- For tumors smaller than 2 cm or well-differentiated tumors, treat GTV + 2 cm margin.
- For tumors 2 cm or larger or poorly differentiated tumors, treat GTV + 2 cm margin + bilateral facial lymphatics ("moustache field") and levels Ib to II bilaterally (Figure 4.7a and b).
- For N+ disease, treat levels I to V bilaterally.
  - CTV (nasal cavity)
    - Treat GTV + 2 cm margin.
    - LN not treated electively if confined to nasal cavity.
    - Tumors that involve superior nasal cavity are often treated with similar field arrangement to maxillary sinus tumor.

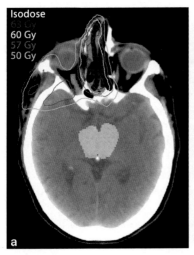

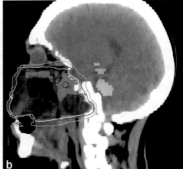

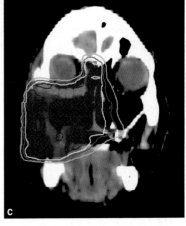

FIGURE 4.6 A 66-year-old woman with T4N0M0 SCC of the R maxillary sinus, s/p endoscopic resection for postoperative radiotherapy to tumor bed only (nodal regions not electively treated). (a) Axial, (b) sagittal, and (c) coronal images displaying isodose distributions. Shaded blue is PTV.

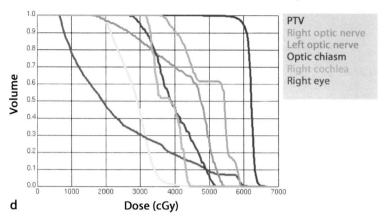

FIGURE 4.6 (Continued) (d) DVH of treatment plan.

Special Considerations

- Fill nasal cavity with wax to reduce dose heterogeneity.
- Interstitial brachytherapy can be used to treat lesions of the nasal septum.
- Cartilage invasion is not a contraindication to definite radiotherapy.

THYROID CANCER

Indications

- Radiotherapy is generally used postoperatively for well-differentiated follicular/papillary cancer that does not take up radioactive iodine if +margin, or +ECE; for all resected anaplastic carcinoma; or for medullary carcinoma that is either locally advanced or associated with an elevated calcitonin level postoperation without evidence of distant disease.

Target Volumes

- CTV (postoperative)
  - Include surgical bed, cervical/SCV/mediastinal nodes at risk.
  - If superior mediastinal nodes are involved, cover entire mediastinum (to subcarinal region). If not, can electively treat superior mediastinum only.
- PTV: per general principles (Figure 4.8a and b).

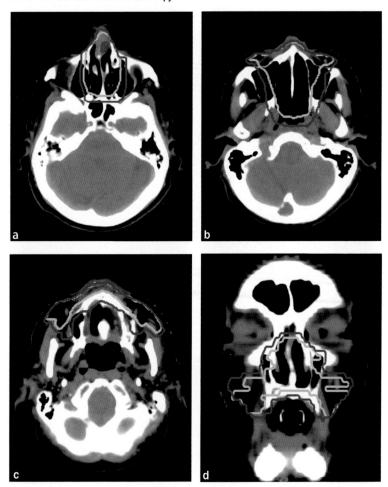

FIGURE 4.7 An 83-year-old woman with a T1N1M0 neuroendocrine carcinoma of the L nasal cavity for definitive radiation. Representative (a-c) axial and (d) coronal images are displayed to demonstrated contours. Shaded red is GTV, thick green line is CTV, and thick blue line is PTV. Note inclusion of facial lymphatics encompassing the region included in traditional "moustache field."

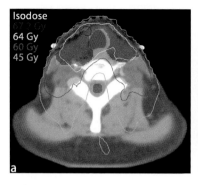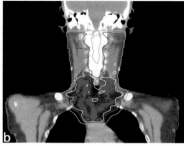

FIGURE 4.8 A 56-year-old woman with recurrent papillary carcinoma of the thyroid, s/p prior thyroidectomy, and radioactive iodine ablation, with bilateral lymphadenopathy and soft tissue disease recurrence, s/p re-resection for postoperative chemoradiation. Representative (a) axial and (b) coronal images displaying isodose distributions. Shaded red is PTV$_{HD}$, shaded blue is PTV$_{ED}$. Note inclusion of upper mediastinal lymphatics.

Special Considerations

- Block oropharynx and oral cavity as much as possible.
- For 3D CRT, often, treatment is AP/posteroanterior initially (42-44 Gy for cord tolerance), then boost tumor bed + ipsilateral neck only with opposed (off cord) obliques.

NONMELANOMATOUS SKIN CANCER

Indications

- Radiotherapy is used in the definitive setting (ie, around nose, ear, and eyelids) for cosmetically superior results, or in the postoperative setting for high-risk or recurrent tumors.

Target Volumes

- GTV (definitive): done clinically
- CTV (definitive)
  - Generally, GTV + 1- to 2-cm margins
  - Use larger margins for more infiltrative or very large lesions.
  - May reduce margin around critical structures (eg, eye and lip).
  - Nodal areas are treated for large, poorly differentiated SCC, or parotid LN +, or N2/3 disease.

- CTV (postoperative): tumor bed + ipsilateral neck nodes + parotid gland (if not removed) + involved named nerves (trigeminal, facial) up to the base of the skull.
- PTV: per general principles.

Special Considerations

- Radiation is delivered with either orthovoltage x-rays (75-125 kVp) or electrons (6-12 MeV). Use skin bolus for electrons. Orthovoltage has its maximum dose at the surface, and less beam constriction at depth. Electrons have sharper dose fall off and are more widely available.
- Use eye shield for eyelid lesions.
- Doses (definitive): greater than 2 Gy dose per fraction is preferred. Frequently used doses include the following: 60 Gy/2.5 Gy/fx, 55 Gy/2.75 Gy/fx, 45 Gy/3 Gy/fx, or 66 to 70 Gy/2 Gy/fx for large tumor abutting critical structures (eg, eye). Doses of 40 Gy/4 Gy/fx, 30 Gy/6 Gy/fx, or 20 Gy/10 Gy/fx are effective regimens when cosmesis is less of a priority.
- Dose (postoperative): standard fractionation 60 Gy to tumor bed and 54 Gy to operative bed and elective nodes. Boost areas of +margin, ECE, PNI.

MELANOMA

Indications

- Radiotherapy is used primarily in the postoperative setting for tumor thickness greater than 4 mm with ulceration or satellite lesions, +margin, N+, or recurrent disease. Desmoplastic histology is controversial.

Target Volumes

- CTV (postoperative): tumor bed + ipsilateral nodal levels II to IV
- PTV: per general principles.

Special Considerations

- Because of the relative radioresistant histology, a higher dose per fraction has been advocated. In the postoperative setting, acceptable regimens include 48 to 50 Gy/2.4 to 2.5 Gy/fx and 60 to 66 Gy/2 to 2.2 Gy/fx for positive margins, +ECE.
- In primary/palliative setting, 30 Gy/6 Gy/fx twice weekly and 50 Gy/2.5 Gy/fx are commonly accepted regimens.
- For melanoma of the scalp, planning options include mixed photon/electron technique versus IMRT versus brachytherapy (6).
- Can consider "sandwiching" bolus material in between 2 thermoplastic masks to ensure consistent setup.

REFERENCES

1. Ahn PH, Garg MK. Positron emission tomography/computed tomography for target delineation in head and neck cancers. *Semin Nucl Med.* 2008;38:141–148.

2. Duan J, Shen S, Spencer SA, et al. A dynamic supraclavicular field-matching technique for head-and-neck cancer patients treated with IMRT. *Int J Radiat Oncol Biol Phys.* 2004;60:959–972.

3. Amdur RJ, Liu C, Li J, Mendenhall W, Hinerman R. Matching intensity-modulated radiation therapy to an anterior low neck field. *Int J Radiat Oncol Biol Phys.* 2007;69:S46–S48.

4. Hansen EK, Bucci MK, Quivey JM, Weinberg V, Xia P. Repeat CT imaging and replanning during the course of IMRT for head-and-neck cancer. *Int J Radiat Oncol Biol Phys.* 2006;64:355–362.

5. Wu Q, Chi Y, Chen PY, Krauss DJ, Yan D, Martinez A. Adaptive replanning strategies accounting for shrinkage in head and neck IMRT. *Int J Radiat Oncol Biol Phys.* 2009;75:924–932.

6. Wojcicka JB, Lasher DE, McAfee SS, Fortier GA. Dosimetric comparison of three different treatment techniques in extensive scalp lesion irradiation. *Radiother Oncol.* 2009;91:255–260.

5 Breast Radiotherapy

Andrew D. Vassil and Rahul D. Tendulkar

GENERAL PRINCIPLES

- Radiation therapy for patients with breast cancer can range from treatment of a tumor bed to chest wall and comprehensive regional nodal radiation fields.
- Patient and disease factors guide the choice of treatment technique.
- Common principles are used when planning radiation therapy, in the setting of both limited and radical surgery.

Localization, Immobilization, and Simulation

- Localization: spiral CT with 3-mm slices spanning the mid-neck to the upper abdomen
- Immobilization: patient is positioned supine or prone (for patients with large or pendulous breast).
  - Cradles, indexed angled breast boards, and prone immobilization devices may be customized to optimize treatment planning.
  - Positioning for external beam radiation is adjusted to limit skin contact at the inframammary sulcus.

- Treatment through the contralateral breast may be avoided by displacing and immobilizing the contralateral breast and by prone positioning techniques.
- Footrests and knee supports help keep patients from sliding down boards. Attaching the breast board to the treatment table makes the immobilization system more rigid, translating into more reproducible treatments.
- Simulation: radiopaque wires are used to delineate target volumes and on all surgical scars.

Target Volumes and Organs of Interest Definition

- Breast: all breast tissue defined clinically and by imaging
- Lumpectomy cavity
  - Included for all patients treated with partial mastectomy

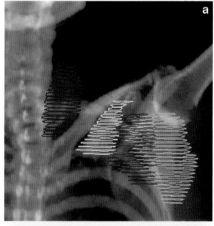
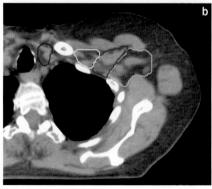

FIGURE 5.1 Lymph node groups displayed on digitally reconstructed AP radiograph (a) and axial image at the level of the proximal clavicle (b). Green indicates level I; blue, level II; yellow, level III; red, SCV lymph nodes.

- Cavity includes seroma and may be determined with the combination of physical examination, CT, ultrasound, and identification of surgical clips (1).
- Chest wall is delineated by landmarks used for external beam breast conservation therapy.
- Lymphatics
  - Delineate nodal groups, heart, and breast tissue
  - Axillary nodal groups are referenced to the pectoralis minor muscle—the level I are lateral, level II are deep, and level III are medial (Figure 5.1).
  - SCV lymph node groups are referenced to the axillary vein.
  - Internal mammary (IM) node fields include the nodes at the first 3 intercostals spaces.

Treatment Planning

- CT–based 3D planning is favored over 2D planning to reduce normal tissue dose and better delineate target areas.
- Segmented and IMRT planning may improve dose homogeneity.

Critical Structures

- Heart: especially relevant to treatment of left-sided breast cancer and IM fields
- 60 Gy to less than one–third of the organ
- 45 Gy to less than two–third of the organ
  - 40 Gy to less than the whole organ
- Lung: especially relevant for SCV fields matched to low breast or chest wall tangent fields
  - V20 to ≤20%

Technical Factors

- 6 MV photons standard
  - Use of higher energy beams may underdose superficial tissues
- Dose homogeneity may be improved by supplementing with 10 MV or higher energy photons and with tissue compensators, including physical wedges, dynamic wedges, segmented field technique (2) and IMRT (3).
- Tumor bed boost fields typically use an en face electron beam.
  - Electron energy selected so that 90% IDL covers tumor bed (CTV) with a 2- to 3-cm expansion
- Dose distribution is calculated with heterogeneity correction
- Optimize plans to result in no more that 5% to 8% dose variation, with maximum dose not exceeding 15% of the prescription

■ Special cases: respiratory gaiting and/or breath-holding techniques may be required to reduce normal tissue doses.

BREAST CONSERVATION—EXTERNAL BEAM RADIOTHERAPY

Introduction

■ Breast conservation techniques include whole-breast and partial-breast radiation.
■ Combinations of multiple photon fields and electron fields are used.

Localization, Immobilization, and Simulation

■ Immobilization: patient is positioned supine on angled breast board (typically 10°-15°) with the ipsilateral hand positioned above the head; the head is rotated toward the contralateral breast.
  ■ Board is angled to make the chest wall parallel to the table, to decrease the amount of collimation used.
  ■ To avoid bolus effect, additional immobilization may be used to limit skin contact at the inframammary sulcus (eg, custom mesh bra or mold).
  ■ Avoiding treatment through the contralateral breast may be accomplished by rotating the gantry and/or displacing and immobilizing the contralateral breast.
■ Simulation: radiopaque wires are placed to delineate tangent fields and on all surgical scars (Figure 5.2).
  ■ Isocenter is placed at least D_{max} depth from surface and typically in a central or deeper location.

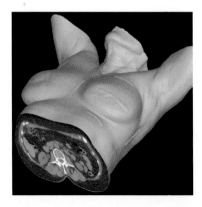

FIGURE 5.2 Simulation—arm above the head with radiopaque wires delineating the target region and scar.

Target Volumes and Organs of Interest Definition

- CTV = residual breast tissue and lumpectomy cavity

Treatment Planning

- Tangent fields
  - Field borders: field borders are delineated with radiopaque wires taped to the skin as follows:
    - Superior: 1 cm above the breast tissue (usually at the inferior aspect of the clavicle or the sternal manubrium joint)
    - Inferior: 2 cm below the inframammary line
    - Medial: mid-sternum
    - Lateral: mid-axillary line
      - Position of the field borders should be modified based on the location of the lumpectomy cavity and areas at higher risk of recurrence.

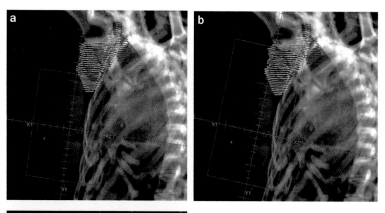

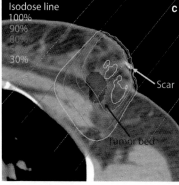

FIGURE 5.3 Standard breast tangent field (a), and "high" breast tangent field (b). Green indicates level I; blue, level II; yellow, level III; red, SCV lymph nodes. Boost field (c) (15 MeV electrons, 100 SSD).

- Medial and lateral tangents: encompass all breast, with posterior edge of beam through medial and lateral radiopaque wires.
  - Rotate the gantry to achieve a flat border posteriorly
  - Rotate the collimator to decrease the amount of lung in field to 3 cm or less (typically 2 cm), flash 2 cm anteriorly (Figure 5.3a)
  - High tangent field with border typically at the level of the humeral head may be considered when electing for additional axillary coverage (Figure 5.3b).
  - Table rotation or a block may be placed at the superior aspect of the tangent fields to reduce divergence into a matched SCV field.
  - Caution when using a heart block for patients with inferiorly located tumors as underdosing of the tumor bed may occur (4).
- Dose homogeneity may be improved with tissue compensators (eg, physical or dynamic wedges).
  - Avoid medial physical wedges owing to concern for scatter radiation dose to the contralateral breast, typically in close proximity to a medial wedge.
  - Segmented field technique may also reduce areas receiving unnecessary high dose.
    - Forward planning is used to manually break the tangent field into multiple segments with reduced field size, essentially blocking portions of the field that are contributing to the high-dose area.
    - IMRT can accomplish a similar effect.
- Boost field
  - The lumpectomy cavity is delineated on planning CT. Ultrasound may aid in delineating the lumpectomy cavity, particularly when the breast tissue is dense and the seroma and/or tumor bed is small (5).
  - En–face field encompassing the scar and lumpectomy cavity with a 2- to 3-cm margin is planned.
  - An electron energy encompassing the lumpectomy cavity with the 80% to 90% isodose line is chosen (typically 9-16 MV electrons; Figure 5.3c).

Dose/Fractionation

- Conventionally, fractionated radiotherapy for whole breast is 45 to 50.4 Gy/1.8 to 2 Gy/fx over approximately 5 weeks.
- Hypofractionated schedules include 42.5 Gy/2.66 Gy/fx daily and 39 Gy/3 Gy/fx every other day (6,7).
  - Typically limited to patients with medial-lateral separation of 25 cm or less (6)
- Boost is typically given as 10 to 16 Gy/2 Gy/fx.

LYMPH NODE RADIOTHERAPY

Introduction

- SCV and IM lymph node radiation is given for patients at higher risk of regional recurrence.
- The main issue with lymph node treatment planning is field matching to breast and chest wall tangent fields.

Localization, Immobilization, and Simulation

- Patient is set up and immobilized as described in the "General Principles" section.
- To match an SCV photon field to breast tangents, 2 techniques may be considered for the tangent fields:
  - Table rotation technique
    - Breast tangent fields are set up as described in the "Breast Conservation—External Beam Radiotherapy" section.
    - For each tangent, the table is rotated away from the gantry to eliminate superior divergence.
  - Half-beam block
    - Isocenter is placed at the superior aspect of what would be the tangent field.
    - A half-beam block is used to eliminate superior divergence.
    - This technique is limited by field size and the inability to rotate the collimator on the tangent fields.

Target Volumes and Organs of Interest Definition

- Use the subclavian vessels and intercostals spaces as reference (8). IV contrast may help delineate nodal regions.
- SCV fields include the high axillary (levels II and III), infraclavicular, and SCV lymph nodes.
- IM lymph node borders
  - Encompass the first 3 intercostal spaces
  - Medial border is the ipsilateral sternal edge or 1 cm medial to the IM vessels if the distance to the sternum is more than 1 cm.
  - The volume extends laterally to include the IM vessels with a 5-mm margin, posteriorly to the pleura, and anteriorly to the anterior extent of the IM vessels (9).

Treatment Planning

- SCV field (Figure 5.4a)
  - Superior: do not flash skin unless inflammatory breast cancer.

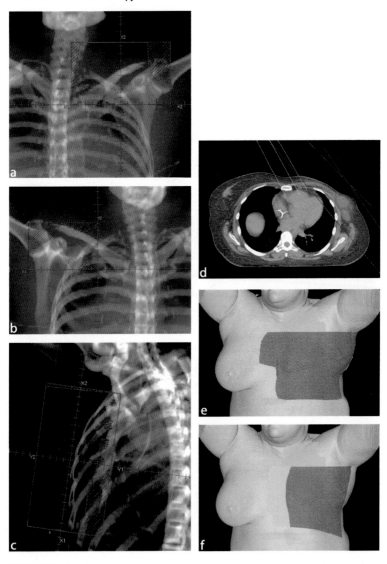

FIGURE 5.4 SCV radiation field (a); posterior axillary boost (b); deep tangent field (c) (IM LN are delineated in red), matched electron IM LN field (d); projection of partially wide tangents (e); and electron field matched to tangents fields (f) used to treat IM LN on a woman after mastectomy. The matched electron field may be separated into multiple fields of different energies to spare deep structures such as heart and lung.

- Inferior: inferior aspect of the clavicular head (this is the level of the iso-center). Placement above the inferior aspect of the clavicular head may result in underdosing of the level III lymph nodes by the SCV field (10).
  - Medial: at pedicles of vertebrae.
  - Lateral: split humeral head; acromioclavicular joint is usually blocked. If specifically targeting the axillary lymph nodes, then consider moving the lateral border lateral to the humeral head; conversely, the lateral border could be placed at the medial aspect of the humeral head if not specifically targeting axillary lymph nodes.
  - Angle the SCV field 10° to 15° off cord by rotating the gantry.
  - Use a half-beam block inferiorly.
  - Prescription is classically to a depth of 3 cm; however, with CT planning, prescribing to the delineated target volumes ensures adequate dose (11).
- Axillary boost field (Figure 5.4 b)
  - PA field used to supplement dose to the mid-axillary plane for patients at high risk of axillary failure.
  - Simulated in the same fashion as an AP SCV field; however, lung blocking is used, and the superior-medial border is moved to the edge of the clavicle.
  - Alternatively, an optimized AP SCV boost field, IMRT may be considered (12).
- IM Fields (Figure 4c-f)
  - Internal mammary lymph nodes are treated by matching a separate field to the tangents or expanding the tangent fields (13). Choice of technique depends on the patient's anatomy and is driven by risk of normal tissue toxicity (9).
  - "Wide" or "deep" tangents include IM nodes by moving the medial border toward the contralateral breast.
  - Partially wide tangents treat the IM nodes and block the heart from the photon field (Figure 5.4c and e). An electron field may supplement dose to the region blocked in the partially wide tangents.
  - An electron field matched to photon tangents is angled to account for the bowing of the isodose distribution (Figure 5.4d and f); the electron field width should be at least 4 cm to allow for adequate dose buildup. A matched photon or mixed photon/electron field (typically 20:80 or 30:70 ratio) may also be considered.

Dose/Fractionation

- SCV field: 45–50 Gy/1.8–2 Gy/fx daily at the start of tangent field radiation.
- Axillary boost field is given simultaneously to bring mid-axillary dose typically to 45 to 50 Gy.
- IM field: 50 Gy/2 Gy/fx daily at the start of tangent field radiation.

BREAST CONSERVATION—PRONE TECHNIQUE

Introduction

- Prone breast techniques aid in delivering radiation therapy to patients with large or pendulous breasts.
- Advantages of prone positioning include the following:
  - Movement of target tissue away from the chest wall
  - Reduced skin folds
  - Reduced lung or heart volume in the radiation field
- Disadvantages of prone positioning include the following:
  - Heart displacement anteriorly (a particular disadvantage for tumor beds near the chest wall)
  - Interference of positioning devices with portal imaging
  - Difficulty visualizing the light fields
  - Inability to treat regional LN

Localization, Immobilization, and Simulation

- The patient is set up prone on a specially designed immobilization device with arms above the head (Figure 5.5a and b).
- The contralateral breast is displaced posteriorly so as not to interfere with the medial tangent field (Figure 5.5c).
- Ipsilateral breast is marked with radiopaque wires as described for supine techniques. Tangential fields are designed as in supine techniques; however, they typically include less lung (often referred to as "lung bite") (Figure 5.5d). Relative to a supine technique, chest wall and breast movement in the prone position is minimal.
- If tumor bed is not accessible for en face boost, repeat simulation in the supine position may be necessary.

Target Volumes and Organs of Interest Definition

- As with supine positioning, fields target breast tissue and lumpectomy CTV.
- As opposed to supine techniques, less lung is typically included in the field. As a result, portions of the chest wall typically may receive less dose. The degree of chest wall included in the treatment field can be adjusted based on the location of the tumor.

Treatment Planning

- Treatment planning principles for prone positioning are the same as those used in supine positioning.

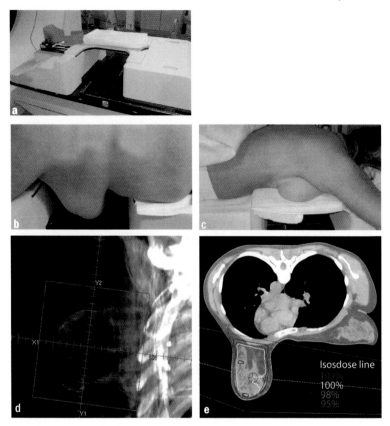

FIGURE 5.5 Prone positioning device (a), patient with cancer of the left breast positioned prone to allow breast tissue to fall anteriorly (b), contralateral breast displaced posteriorly (c), typical treatment port (d), and isodose distribution achieved (e) for a patient for whom dose was prescribed to the 98% IDL using 6 MV photons, field-within-field technique, no wedges.

- The main dosimetric advantage is a decreased skin fold at the inframammary sulcus and decreased separation from entrance to exit.
- Chest wall and lung receive less dose than would be expected in a supine position (Figure 5.5e).

Dose/Fractionation

- Dose and fractionation for prone positioning are the same as those used in supine positioning.

BREAST CONSERVATION—ACCELERATED PARTIAL BREAST RADIOTHERAPY

Introduction

- Balloon catheter brachytherapy, multicatheter interstitial brachytherapy, intraoperative techniques, and 3D conformal external beam RT using photon or electron fields are the predominant treatment techniques.
- Only balloon catheter brachytherapy technique will be discussed here, based on the NSABP B-39/RTOG 0413 protocol.

Simulation

- Balloon is placed in lumpectomy cavity at the time of surgery or postoperatively under ultrasound guidance.
- Balloon is filled with saline (30-70 mL) mixed with 1 to 2 mL contrast.
- Patient is positioned supine with the ipsilateral hand positioned above the head; the head is rotated toward the contralateral breast.
- Computed tomography images from mandible to several centimeters below the inframammary sulcus (inclusive of entire lung) are produced.

Target Volumes and Organs of Interest Definition

- PTV: 10 mm circumferential expansion around the balloon, less the balloon volume. Regions 5 mm from the skin surface and area of the chest wall/pectoralis muscles are excluded from PTV.
- Air and fluid trapped around the balloon are delineated.

Treatment Planning

- Tissue-balloon conformance: %PTV coverage – [(vol trapped air/vol PTV) × 100] should equal 90% or higher. Adequate PTV coverage cannot be achieved if this value is less than 90% if the percentage of PTV displaced is greater than 10%. Ninety percent or greater of the prescribed dose should cover 90% or greater of the PTV.
- Balloon symmetry: balloon geometry should be within 2 mm of expected dimensions.
- Minimal balloon surface-skin distance: 7 mm or greater is optimal; however, 5 to 7 mm is acceptable. Skin dose maximum is 145% or lower of prescription dose (Figure 5.6).
- Normal tissue dose volume parameters: volume of tissue receiving 150% (V150) and 200% (V200) of the prescribed dose is limited to 50 cc or lower and 10 cc or lower, respectively.
- Uninvolved normal breast: less than 60% of the whole-breast volume should receive 50% or greater of the prescribed dose. Balloon volume is subtracted from the breast volume.

Dose/fractionation

- Brachytherapy: HDR: 34 Gy/10fx prescribed at 1 cm from the balloon surface. Treatments are delivered BID over 5 to 7 days with an interfraction interval of 6 hours or more.
- 3DCRT: 38.5 Gy/3.85 Gy/fx delivered BID over 5 to 7 days with an interfraction interval of 6 hours or more.

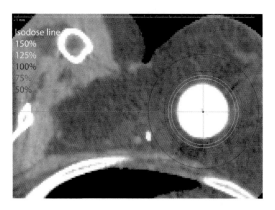

FIGURE 5.6 Woman with a brachytherapy balloon catheter in place; 50% to 150% isodose lines from ^{192}Ir source are displayed.

POSTMASTECTOMY RADIOTHERAPY

Introduction

- Postmastectomy radiotheraphy includes chest wall treatments and may extend to target nodal regions.
- Combinations of photon and electron fields may be used to individualize treatments.
- Techniques include standard tangents (±matched IM node fields), electron fields, wide tangents, and partially wide tangent fields. A "reverse hockey stick" technique involves AP/PA photon fields treating the SCV lymph nodes and lateral chest wall matched to a medial electron field targeting the medial chest wall and IM lymph nodes (this will not be discussed in this section).
- Immediate breast reconstruction is discouraged when postmastectomy radiotherapy is part of an overall treatment plan (14).
  - Coverage of IM lymph nodes is often compromised
  - Tangent angle selection can be impacted
  - Flexibility of electron-only chest wall treatment is eliminated

Localization, Immobilization, and Simulation

- The patient is set up in a supine position on a breast board and CT scan is conducted as described in the "General Principles" section.
- Contralateral breast tissue or measurements made prior to radical surgery may be used to delineate the superior, inferior, medial, and lateral field dimensions (particularly for patients with inflammatory breast cancer and those who have undergone bilateral mastectomy).
- Similar landmarks to those used in breast conservation are delineated with radiopaque wire taped to the skin (inferior aspect of clavicular head, midsternum, mid-axillary line, 2 cm below the level of the contralateral inframammary sulcus).
- Photon tangents (Figure 5.7a)
  - Medial and lateral tangents are designed with posterior edge of beam through medial and lateral radiopaque wires.
  - Blocking and table rotation are used to reduce divergence into a matched SCV field.
  - The medial border may be moved toward the contralateral breast/chest wall to provide additional coverage of IM lymph nodes (ie, wide or partially wide tangents, see "Lymph Node radiotherapy" section).
  - Isocenter is placed at least D_{max} from the skin surface for photon tangent fields.
- Electron fields (Figure 5.7b)
  - After delineation of the chest wall target volume, the field is broken into multiple en face fields (typically 2 fields).
  - Isocenter for each field located at the skin surface.
- Boost field: en face electrons encompassing the scar with 3- to 5-cm margin, using energy sufficient for the 90% IDL to encompass the surface to chest wall thickness (Figure 5.7c).
- Description of matching nodal fields is described in the "Lymph node radiotherapy" section.

Target Volumes and Organs of Interest Definition

- CTV = the entire chest wall (skin surface to rib-soft tissue interface)
  - IM nodes are typically included although not specifically targeted unless disease factors warrant doing so.
  - Ipsilateral SCV volumes should be delineated if they are to be targeted.
- A scar boost may be considered if there is high risk of local recurrence (eg, positive or close margins and inflammatory breast cancer).
- Lung and heart volumes are delineated.

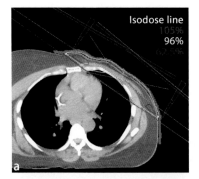

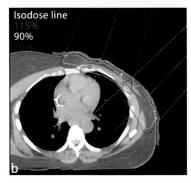

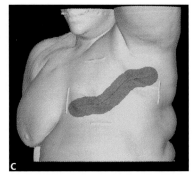

FIGURE 5.7 Isodose distribution from tangent photon fields (a) and matched electron fields (b). Mixed 6 and 10 MV photons with 25° wedges prescribed to the 96% isodose line using 5 mm tissue equivalent bolus were used for the photon fields. A medial field of 9 MV electrons and a lateral field of 12 MV electrons, 100 SSD at skin surface using 5-mm tissue equivalent bolus were used for the electron fields. A en face boost with a 3 cm radial margin on the mastectomy scar was designed for an electron boost (c).

Treatment Planning

- 3- to 5-mm of tissue-equivalent bolus material may be applied at the time of simulation or modeled with virtual simulation.
- For inflammatory breast cancer patients and others, bolus may be applied daily at the beginning of treatment and titrated to effect with the goal of brisk erythema at the completion of therapy. Sample schedules of bolus used include the following:
  - 5 mm bolus daily during weeks 1 and 2, every other day during weeks 3 and 4, then off

- 3 mm bolus daily during weeks 1 to 3, then every other day until treatment is completed
- Clinical judgment must be used when determining duration of bolus use.
- Dose heterogeneity corrections should be applied unless artifact because metal components in tissue expanders are present.
- Photon tangents
  - Treatments are typically prescribed to the 95% isodose line.
  - Optimized dose homogeneity may require tissue compensators (eg, physical wedges, dynamic wedges, and IMRT).
  - Standard tangents typically have less coverage of IM nodes; however, a lower V20 is usually achieved.
  - Partially wide tangents to treat the IM nodes may help reduce dose to the heart.
- Electron fields
  - Overlapping fields, also known as "hot matching," may be done to ensure adequate coverage of junctions; however, a noticeable match-line fibrosis may result.
  - Junction shifts of 0.5 cm every 5 fractions may be used to reduce the risk for match-line fibrosis.
  - Electron energy is selected such that the 90% IDL encompasses the chest wall thickness to the anterior pleural surface (typically 6-12 MV electrons); this would also serve as the prescription isodose line.

Dose/Fractionation

- Chest wall fields deliver 45 to 50.4/1.8 to 2 Gy/fx daily.
- Boost field delivers 10 to 16 Gy/2 Gy/fx.
- Supraclavicular region is treated to 46 to 50 Gy/2 Gy/fx.
- Inflammatory breast cancer: consider 1.5 Gy per fx BID ($\geq$6-hour interfraction interval) to 51 Gy delivered to the chest wall and regional nodes, followed by a 15-Gy boost to the chest wall with electrons. Brisk erythema at the completion of treatment is desirable.

- The mid-axilla may be supplemented in high risk cases (see "SCV lymph node radiotherapy").

REFERENCES

1. Goldberg H, Prosnitz RG, Olson JA, Marks LB. Definition of postlumpectomy tumor bed for radiotherapy boost field planning: CT versus surgical clips. *Int J Radiat Oncol Biol Phys.* 2005;63:209–213.

2. Ludwig V, Schwab F, Guckenberger M, Krieger T, Flentje M. Comparison of wedge versus segmented techniques in whole breast irradiation: effects on dose exposure outside the treatment volume. *Strahlenther Onkol.* 2008;184:307–312.

3. Descovich M, Fowble B, Bevan A, Schechter N, Park C, Xia P. Comparison between hybrid direct aperture optimized intensity-modulated radiotherapy and forward planning intensity-modulated radiotherapy for whole breast irradiation. *Int J Radiat Oncol Biol Phys.* 2009.

4. Raj KA, Evans ES, Prosnitz RG, et al. Is there an increased risk of local recurrence under the heart block in patients with left-sided breast cancer? *Cancer J.* 2006;12:309–317.

5. Berrang TS, Truong PT, Popescu C, et al. 3D ultrasound can contribute to planning CT to define the target for partial breast radiotherapy. *Int J Radiat Oncol Biol Phys.* 2009;73:375–383.

6. Whelan T, MacKenzie R, Julian J, et al. Randomized trial of breast irradiation schedules after lumpectomy for women with lymph node–negative breast cancer. *J Natl Cancer Inst.* 2002;94:1143–1150.

7. Bentzen SM, Agrawal RK, Aird EG, et al. The UK Standardisation of Breast Radiotherapy (START) Trial A of radiotherapy hypofractionation for treatment of early breast cancer: a randomised trial. *Lancet Oncol.* 2008;9:331–341.

8. Madu CN, Quint DJ, Normolle DP, Marsh RB, Wang EY, Pierce LJ. Definition of the supraclavicular and infraclavicular nodes: implications for three-dimensional CT-based conformal radiation therapy. *Radiology* 2001;221:333–339.

9. Pierce LJ, Butler JB, Martel MK, et al. Postmastectomy radiotherapy of the chest wall: dosimetric comparison of common techniques. *Int J Radiat Oncol Biol Phys* 2002;52:1220–1230.

10. Garg AK, Frija EK, Sun TL, et al. Effects of variable placement of superior tangential/supraclavicular match line on dosimetric coverage of level III axilla/axillary apex in patients treated with breast and supraclavicular radiotherapy. *Int J Radiat Oncol Biol Phys.* 2009;73:370–374.

11. Liengsawangwong R, Yu TK, Sun TL, et al. Treatment optimization using computed tomography–delineated targets should be used for supraclavicular irradiation for breast cancer. *Int J Radiat Oncol Biol Phys.* 2007;69:711–715.

12. Wang X, Yu TK, Salehpour M, Zhang SX, Sun TL, Buchholz TA. Breast cancer regional radiation fields for supraclavicular and axillary lymph node treatment: is a posterior axillary boost field technique optimal? *Int J Radiat Oncol Biol Phys.* 2009;74:86–91.

13. Arthur DW, Arnfield MR, Warwicke LA, Morris MM, Zwicker RD. Internal mammary node coverage: an investigation of presently accepted techniques. *Int J Radiat Oncol Biol Phys*. 2000;48:139–146.

14. Motwani SB, Strom EA, Schechter NR, et al. The impact of immediate breast reconstruction on the technical delivery of postmastectomy radiotherapy. *Int J Radiat Oncol Biol Phys*. 2006;66:76–82.

6 Thoracic Radiotherapy

Grant K. Hunter and Gregory M. M. Videtic

GENERAL PRINCIPLES

- General principles for planning thoracic radiotherapy (TRT) are valid across a range of malignancies and include simulation techniques, definition of dose-limiting structures, dose constraints, and beam setups.
- Specific dose prescriptions are determined by tumor types and treatment approaches, whether preoperative, definitive, or postoperative therapy.

Localization, Immobilization, and Simulation

- Volumetric treatment planning (computed tomography [CT] simulation on a flat surface) for definition of gross tumor volume (GTV), clinical tumor volume (CTV), and planning target volume (PTV)
- Patient position: supine
- Immobilization: generally arms raised above the head
  - Pancoast tumor may require arms akimbo.
  - Numerous different systems (eg, vacuum-type immobilization bag and thermoplastic mold) are commercially available to position the arms above the head in a reproducible, patient-friendly manner.
- Localization: contiguous spiral CT slices acquired with 3-mm slice acquisition through the chest from the level of the cricoid cartilage inferiorly to include the whole liver.

- Contrast agents
  - Oral contrast to delineate esophagus.
  - As needed, intravenous contrast to delineate major blood vessels.
- Treatment planning FDG-PET/CT scan with the patient in treatment position is desirable.
  - Otherwise, staging PET done prior to simulation may be coregistered with simulation CT for contouring, mindful of positional and table differences.
- Target motion
  - Tumor motion due to respiration must be taken into account during treatment planning. There are a range of valid approaches (see details in "Tools for Simulation and Treatment"):
    - 4-dimensional CT
    - Physical control/restriction of tumor motion
    - Gating/fiducials
    - Free breathing

Target Volumes and Organs of Interest

- Reference should be made to the 1993 International Commission on Radiation Units & Measurements report 62 document for a complete description of the various target volume definitions (GTV, CTV, and PTV).
- Normal anatomy to be routinely identified
  - Lungs: right and left done separately, then combined as a composite lung volume.
  - Heart: from its base (RTOG definition: beginning at the CT slice where the ascending aorta originates and encompassing the great vessels) to the apex.
  - Esophagus: from the bottom of the cricoid to the gastroesophageal junction.
  - Spinal cord: the spinal cord should be contoured on each CT slice.
  - Brachial plexus, liver, kidneys: as needed, based on tumor location.

Treatment Planning

- 3D conformal therapy: contemporary outcomes by and large based on TRT planning with combinations of coplanar or noncoplanar 3D conformal fields, without heterogeneity corrections or accounting for tumor motion.
- IMRT: thoracic IMRT is increasingly being used in chest treatment. In the setting of IMRT, clinicians must be able to control respiratory motion to limit excursion.
  - The National Cancer Institute-published "Guidelines for the Use of IMRT" can be found on the following Web site: http://www.qarc.org/Protocols/IMRTGuidelines.pdf.

Critical Structures

- Normal tissue constraints are prioritized in the following order by importance for treatment planning:
  - Spinal cord: highest priority dose constraint, irrespective of other constraints.
    - Total (direct plus scatter) dose must not exceed 50.5 Gy (point dose within spinal cord).
  - Lung: the volume of *both* lungs that receives more than 20 Gy (the V20) should not exceed 37% of the total. Alternatively, the mean lung dose should optimally be 20 Gy or less.
    - Total lung volume = combined lungs minus the CTV.
  - Esophagus: mean dose to the esophagus is optimally kept below 34 Gy but is not an absolute requirement. Keeping V55 below 33% is also an alternative constraint.
  - Heart
    - 60 Gy to less than one third of the organ
    - 45 Gy to less than two thirds of the organ
    - 40 Gy to less than the whole organ
  - Brachial plexus (for tumors in mid/upper thorax): ≤60 Gy.

Technical Factors

Beam energies

- Photon energies: 6 to 10 MV; higher energy photons (>10 MV) are not recommenced in lung tissue as the beam penumbra increases and the beam edge becomes less sharp. Also, for higher energy photons (>10 MV), the prescribed dose at the periphery of the tumor may be decreased, more so with small fields, so higher energy beams are to be avoided.

Beam shaping

- Multileaf collimation or individually shaped (5 HVL) custom blocks for normal tissue protection outside the target volume.

Heterogeneity corrections

- Historically, TRT plans used "uncorrected" dose calculations that replace all body tissue by a water equivalent, that is, homogeneous dose deposition in tissues assuming homogenous tissue electron densities.
- Currently, TRT now distinguishes the heterogeneous nature of tissues in the chest to more appropriately predict dose, dose deposition, normal tissue toxicities, and outcomes. Therefore, heterogeneity corrections are now

recommended in general treatment planning (see section on "Helpful Physics Facts" for depiction of heterogeneity correction).

NON–SMALL CELL LUNG CANCER

TRT Indications

- Definitive TRT with concurrent chemotherapy is the standard of care for patients with stage III unresectable non–small cell lung cancer (NSCLC) and selected inoperable stage II patients.
- Preoperative or postoperative TRT may be indicated in selected stage II or III NSCLC patients.

Target Volume Definitions

A. Definitive TRT (see Figure 6.1)

- GTV = primary tumor + clinically positive nodes seen on planning CT (>1 cm short axis diameter) or pretreatment PET scan (SUV >3)
  - Contour primary tumor using "lung windows" setting.
  - The volumes may be disjointed or noncontinuous.

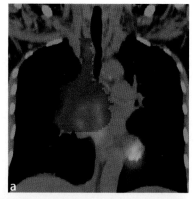

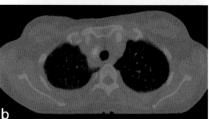

FIGURE 6.1 A 53-year-old woman with T3N2M0 NSCLC of the right upper lobe, treated definitively with concurrent chemoradiotherapy. Diagnostic PET fused to CT simulation images to aid in planning target volumes. Coronal (a) and axial (b) planning CT and diagnostic PET images coregistered, with GTV depicted in red.

- In the event of a collapsed lobe/lung segment, use PET to distinguish tumor from fluid/atelectasis.
- CTV = GTV + 0.5 to 1 cm margin to account for microscopic extension.
  - Pathologic studies suggest microscopic extension a function, of histologic subtype.
  - If an ITV is used then, the CTV = ITV + 0.5 to 1 cm.
  - Elective nodal irradiation (ENI).
    - Until recently, standard TRT practice in the United States has been to deliver dose electively to nonclinically involved regional hilar, mediastinal, and/or supraclavicular nodal areas.
    - Modern imaging techniques (especially PET) and studies of nodal failure patterns have shifted practice away from ENI to including only grossly involved or high-risk nodal basins in the target.
    - Remains an area of investigation.
- PTV.
  - For breath hold or gating (non-ITV) approach
    - PTV margin = CTV +1 cm in the superior/inferior direction and 0.5 cm in the axial plane, with daily imaging.
  - For ITV approach
    - PTV = CTV + 1 cm, unless daily imaging is used, then setup margins may be reduced to 0.5 cm.
  - For free-breathing, non-ITV approach
    - PTV = CTV+ 1.5 cm superior/inferior and at least 1 cm in axial plane.

B. Preoperative RT (Figure 6.2a and b)

- GTV, CTV, PTV: per definitions used in section A above
- Consider
  - Inclusion of nodal stations adjacent to involved nodes.
  - Any nodal stations connecting involved stations when skip metastases are present.

C. Postoperative TRT (Figure 6.2c and d)

- Reference preoperative imaging (CT and PET) and investigations for primary tumor and involved nodal (GTV) localization and boundaries
- CTV should include, at a minimum,
  - Bronchial stump
  - Ipsilateral hilum
  - Pathologically involved nodal stations
  - Consider
    - Inclusion of nodal stations adjacent to involved nodes.

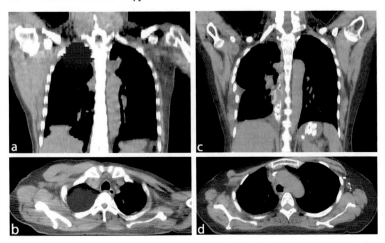

FIGURE 6.2 Coronal (a) and axial (b) images from a 63-year-old man with a Pancoast tumor (NSCLC) involving the right upper lobe (RUL) treated preoperatively (GTV in red). Coronal (c) and axial (d) images from a 44-year-old woman with resected NSCLC stage III (T2N2M0) of the right lower lobe (CTV in green).

- • Any nodal stations connecting involved stations when skip metastases are present.
- ■ CTV for positive margins/extracapsular extension should reference
  - ■ Preoperative GTVs
  - ■ Surgical clips
  - ■ Operative reports

Treatment Planning

Dose/Fractionation
- ■ A. Definitive TRT: conventional therapy is 60 to 66 Gy/1.8 to 2 Gy/fx
  - ■ Figure 6.3 is a representative DVH for a patient receiving definitive radiation.
- ■ B. Preoperative RT: 45 to 50.4 Gy/1.8 to 2Gy/fx followed by surgery at 4 to 6 weeks
- ■ C. Postoperative TRT: 45 to 60 Gy/1.8 to 2 Gy/fx as a function of nodal and margin status

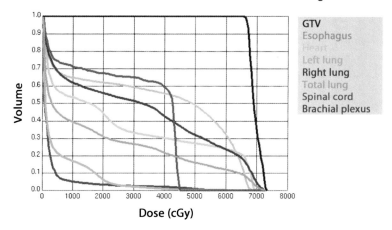

FIGURE 6.3 DVH for definitive TRT in stage III NSCLC: 64 Gy/2 Gy/fx, 3-field technique, 10 MV photons prescribed to the 96% isodose line.

SMALL CELL LUNG CANCER

TRT Indications

- "Early start" TRT (with cycles 1 or 2 of chemotherapy (1,2)) is recommended for definitive treatment of limited stage disease.

Target Volumes Definitions

- GTV = primary tumor and involved nodes (PET positive or >1-1.5 cm in diameter on CT).
- CTV = GTV + 1.5 to 2 cm margin
  - Elective nodal irradiation (see NSCLC for review).
    - Elective nodal irradiation remains controversial but is generally not recommended.
- PTV = 0.5 to 1 cm expansion of CTV, per tumor control technique.
- Special Considerations.
  - TRF after chemotherapy impacts on target definition.
  - In patients with radiographic complete response after full chemotherapy treatment, ipsilateral hilum/mediastinum should be treated.
  - When TRT is delayed after chemotherapy, the use of larger field pre-chemotherapy volumes versus smaller postchemotherapy volumes is somewhat controversial, with postchemotherapy volumes preferred (3).

Dose/Fractionation

- 45 Gy/1.5 Gy/fx twice daily (4).
- Alternative schedules: 50 to 70 Gy/1.8 to 2 Gy/fx from nonrandomized trials.

THYMOMA

TRT Indications

- TRT for thymoma is most commonly used in the adjuvant setting. Also indicated for thymic carcinomas.
- Definitive TRT (+/- chemotherapy) for medically inoperable or surgically unresectable patients.

Target Volume Definitions

- Use preoperative imaging to reference tumor location and fuse to simulation CT images for target definition.
- GTV = generally not applicable, note surgical clips and relations to preoperative tumor.
- CTV = surgical bed/resected volume, generally no nodal targets.
- PTV = CTV + 1 cm, target motion minimal.

Treatment Planning

- Classical field arrangements for resected thymoma are a "wedged pair" or anteroposterior/posteroanterior fields with anterior weighting (Figure 6.4).

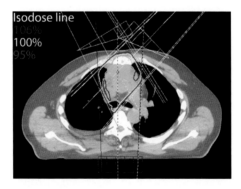

FIGURE 6.4 Axial planning CT image from a 56-year-old man with resected Masaoka stage II thymoma, WHO type C; postoperative TRT, 60 Gy/2 Gy/fx, 3-field plan with wedged 6 and 10 MV photons.

Dose/Fractionation

- For adjuvant TRT: 45 to 50 Gy for negative margins
- 54 to 60 Gy for microscopically positive margins
- 60 to 66 Gy for gross/residual disease
- 2 Gy fraction size recommended

ESOPHAGEAL CARCINOMA

TRT Indications

- The role of TRT in the definitive management of esophageal cancer is controversial.
- Preoperative, definitive, and postoperative TRT are all advocated, depending on institutional and clinician preference.
- Cervical esophageal carcinomas have historically been judged unresectable and treated with definitive TRT +/- chemotherapy.

Special Considerations at Simulation

- For cervical and upper third thoracic lesions, immobilization with a mask is preferred.
- Oral contrast and intravenous contrast may improve visualization of the esophageal mass or strictures to help with contouring. In the postoperative setting, oral contrast is not given.
- There is currently no defined role for motion compensating techniques.

Target Volume Definitions

Definitive TRT (see Figure 6.5a)

- GTV = gross tumor and PET positive regional lymph nodes
- CTV = GTV + 4 cm proximal and distal and + 1 cm radially
- PTV = CTV+ 1 to 2 cm proximally and distally and + 1 cm radially

Preoperative /postoperative TRT

- Essentially replicates definitive fields.
- Use CT and PET imaging to define primary and nodal target boundaries (Figure 6.5b and c).

Dose/Fractionation

- Definitive TRT: 50.4 Gy/1.8 Gy/fx
  - The use of brachytherapy boost in the definitive setting is controversial (5).

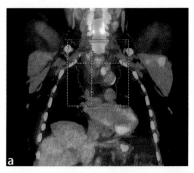

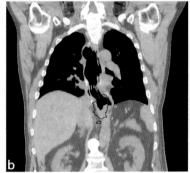

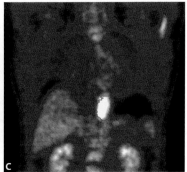

FIGURE 6.5 (a) Coronal image from a 78-year-old man, definitive TRT for cervical esophageal cancer, 64 Gy/2 Gy/fx; planning CT images coregistered to diagnostic PET images (CTV in red). (b) A 63-year-old man, resected stage III esophageal cancer, postoperative TRT, 50.4 Gy/1.8 Gy/fx, with concurrent chemotherapy. Coronal CT planning image with CTV in red. (c) Preoperative PET scan was fused to the postoperative CT simulation scan in order to aid in target delineation. Target contour in red.

■ Preoperative TRT: dose ranges from 40 to 50.4 Gy/1.8 to 2 Gy/fx.
■ Postoperative radiation dose: 45 to 50.4 Gy/1.8 to 2 Gy/fx (6,7).

MESOTHELIOMA

TRT Indications

■ Definitive TRT is indicated adjuvantly after extrapleural pneumonectomy (EPP).

Special Considerations at Simulation

■ Visualize incision/drainage sites with radiopaque material.

- Consider bolus on the chest wall to ensure adequate dose delivery to the scar or any drain sites, with a 2- to 4-cm margin.

Target Volume Definition (Figure 6.6a-c)

- Surgical clips aid in the delineation of medial pre-resected diaphragm, inferior diaphragm insertion, and sternopericardial recess.
- GTV = not applicable
- CTV = all potential pleura-bearing surfaces from the involved lung, including the chest wall from the apex to the lung bases, pericardium, diaphragmatic crural insertions, any surgical mesh reconstruction, ipsilateral hilum, and mediastinal boundary, with inclusion of all surgical clips.
  - Particular attention is to be paid to identifying and contouring the posterior and inferior aspects of the insertions of the diaphragm, for inclusion in the CTV.

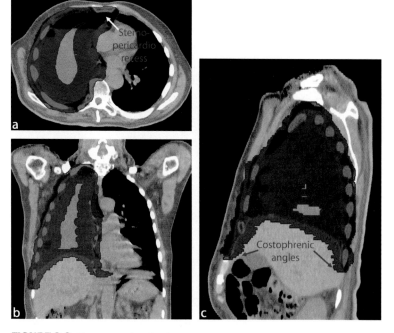

FIGURE 6.6 Treatment planning images for a 70-year-old man with a pT2N0M0 malignant mesothelioma post-EPP; adjuvant TRT, 54 Gy/2 Gy/fx; IMRT, 10 MV photons. Axial (a), coronal (b), and sagittal (c) images are shown, with PTV depicted in blue. Note the costophrenic angles and sternopericardial recess.

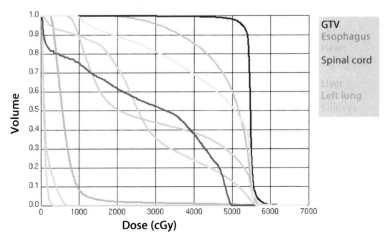

FIGURE 6.7 Dose-volume histogram for the IMRT plan of the patient receiving 54 Gy after EPP depicted in Figure 6.6.

- Boost volumes
  - Ipsilateral mediastinum in the setting of resected N2 disease
  - Positive margins/gross residual disease
- PTV = CTV + 5- to 8-mm expansion

TABLE 6.1 IMRT recommendations for Post-EPP TRT

Target or Organ	Dose Goal or Constraint Dose
PTV (CTV+ 5-7 mm)	≥ 95% coverage with 54 Gy
Intact lung	<20% to receive >20 Gy; <60% to receive >5 Gy; mean lung dose ≤10 Gy
Liver	<30% to receive >30 Gy
Kidney	<20% to receive >15 Gy
Heart	<50% to receive >45 Gy
Spinal cord	<10% to receive >45 Gy; no portion to receive >50 Gy
Esophagus	<30% to receive >55 Gy; mean dose ≤34 Gy

Abbreviation: IMRT, intensity-modulated radiation therapy.

Dose/Fractionation

- 54 Gy/2 Gy/fx to ipsilateral hemithorax Gy for positive margins/gross disease.

Planning considerations (see DVH; Figure 6.7)

- Intensity-modulated radiation therapy is recommended in the setting of adjuvant mesothelioma (Table 6.1; 8–9).
  - Mean lung dose of intact lung <10 Gy.

STEREOTACTIC BODY RADIOTHERAPY FOR LUNG TUMORS

Stereotactic Body RT Indications

- Medically inoperable T1/T2N0M0 NSCLC
- Oligometastatic disease to the lungs in selected patients

Special Considerations at Simulation

- Rigid immobilization.
- Tumor range of motion to be kept to less than 1 cm (methods as detailed in "General Principles, Tumor Motion").

Target Volume Definitions

- GTV = Lung lesion, as drawn using CT images on "lung windows" setting
- CTV = GTV
- ITV = target representing the range of GTV motion through the breathing cycle (see Figure 6.8)
- PTV = CTV + 3- to 10-mm margin; expansion will reflect the parameters of the particular delivery system, tumor motion control paradigm, and dose planning algorithm for any given institution

Treatment Planning

- North American collaborative group standard set by RTOG 0236 protocol
- May include 3D, IMRT, helical-based approaches
- General goals of planning
  - Delineation of all normal thoracic structures
  - All organs at risk to have detailed dose constraints, defined both by maximum point dose and by volume
  - Dose constraints will vary by fractionation schedules.
  - Coverage of at least 95% of the PTV by prescription isodose curve, with tight control of dose spillage around the target

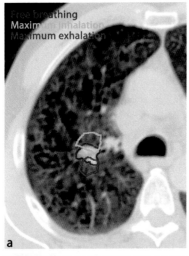

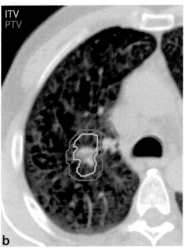

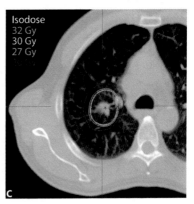

FIGURE 6.8 A 57-year-old man with medically inoperable NSCLC of the right upper lobe, treated on an SBRT protocol: 30 Gy/1 fx. (a) From the CT simulation, this image depicts the GTV during free breathing (red), at maximum inhalation (green), and maximum exhalation (blue). (b) ITV (lime) was generated by combining GTVs. PTV (light blue) = ITV + 5 mm. Isodose distribution using a 6-arc plan, 6 MV photons, prescribed to the 80% isodose line (c).

Dose/Fractionation

■ RTOG 0236 schedule: 60 Gy/20 Gy/fx over 8 to 14 days; other regimens frequently used: 48 Gy/12 Gy/fx and 50 Gy/10 Gy/fx.

REFERENCES

1. Jeremic B, Shibamoto Y, Acimovic L, et al: Initial versus delayed accelerated hyperfractionated radiation therapy and concurrent chemotherapy in

limited small-cell lung cancer: a randomized study. *J Clin Oncol*. 1997;15: 893–900.

2. Murray N, Coy P, Pater JL, et al: Importance of timing for thoracic irradiation in the combined modality treatment of limited-stage small-cell lung cancer. The National Cancer Institute of Canada Clinical Trials Group. *J Clin Oncol*. 1993;11:336–344.

3. Kies MS, Mira JG, Crowley JJ, et al: Multimodal therapy for limited small-cell lung cancer: a randomized study of induction combination chemotherapy with or without thoracic radiation in complete responders; and with wide-field versus reduced-field radiation in partial responders: a Southwest Oncology Group Study. *J Clin Oncol*. 1987;5:592–600.

4. Turrisi AT, 3rd, Kim K, Blum R, et al: Twice-daily compared with once-daily thoracic radiotherapy in limited small-cell lung cancer treated concurrently with cisplatin and etoposide. *N Engl J Med*. 1999;340:265–271.

5. Gaspar LE, Winter K, Kocha WI, et al: A phase I/II study of external beam radiation, brachytherapy, and concurrent chemotherapy for patients with localized carcinoma of the esophagus (Radiation Therapy Oncology Group Study 9207): final report. *Cancer* 2000;88:988–995.

6. Macdonald JS, Smalley SR, Benedetti J, et al: Chemoradiotherapy after surgery compared with surgery alone for adenocarcinoma of the stomach or gastroesophageal junction. *N Engl J Med*. 2001;345:725–730.

7. Bedard EL, Inculet RI, Malthaner RA, et al: The role of surgery and postoperative chemoradiation therapy in patients with lymph node positive esophageal carcinoma. *Cancer* 2001;91:2423–2430.

8. Forster KM, Smythe WR, Starkschall G, et al: Intensity-modulated radiotherapy following extrapleural pneumonectomy for the treatment of malignant mesothelioma: clinical implementation. *Int J Radiat Oncol Biol Phys*. 2003;55:606–616.

9. Ahamad A, Stevens CW, Smythe WR, et al: Intensity-modulated radiation therapy: a novel approach to the management of malignant pleural mesothelioma. *Int J Radiat Oncol Biol Phys*. 2003;55:768–775.

10. Miles EF, Larrier NA, Kelsey CR, et al: Intensity-modulated radiotherapy for resected mesothelioma: the Duke experience. *Int J Radiat Oncol Biol Phys*. 2008;71:1143–1150.

7 Gastrointestinal (Non-esophageal) Radiotherapy

Michael J. Burdick and Kevin L. Stephans

GENERAL PRINCIPLES

- General principles relevant to EBRT planning of gastrointestinal (GI) malignancies include simulation techniques, definition of dose-limiting structures, dose constraints, and planning principles.
- Specific dose prescription will be determined by tumor types and treatment approaches, for example, preoperative, definitive, or postoperative therapy.

Localization, Immobilization, and Simulation

- Volumetric treatment planning (CT simulation on a flat surface) for the definition of GTV, CTV, and PTV.
- Patient position: specific to tumor site and stage.
- Immobilization: arms raised above the head. A range of immobilization systems are available. The use of a "belly board" for small bowel displacement may be appropriate for a range of GI malignancies.
- Contiguous spiral CT slices acquired with 3- to 5-mm slice acquisition.

- For pancreas and stomach tumors, obtain images from above the diaphragm to below the kidneys.
- For rectal and anal cancers, obtain images from the L3 vertebral body to 6 in. below an external anal marker.
- Contrast agents and fiducial/tumor markers
  - Oral contrast is used to delineate the small bowel. One should allow a 2-hour transit time for the agent through the small bowel.
  - IV contrast to delineate the tumor and LN; alternatively, may fuse contrasted diagnostic CT scan to the planning images.
  - Barium enema may help delineate rectal and anal tumors.
    - This will influence the use of heterogeneity corrections in treatment planning and may displace the tumor.
    - If contrast is used, a scan without contrast should also be obtained to define a lesion's "natural" position and to aid with heterogeneity collections.
  - For rectal and anal malignancies, a marker at the level of the anus aids the determination of the inferior field borders.
  - In post-surgical patients, the location of surgical clips matched to preoperative imaging can aid in the delineation of the resected tumor bed.
    - NB: surgery alters normal anatomy, so clips should be used for reference only.
    - Clip placement may not reflect tumor location, for example, hemostasis clip versus tumor resection margin.

Target Volumes and Organs of Interest Definition

- Reference should be made to the 1993 ICRU report 62 document for complete description of various target volume definitions (GTV, CTV, and PTV).
- Normal anatomy to be routinely identified for pancreas/gastric cancer
  - Liver
  - Small bowel
  - Kidneys
  - Spinal cord
- Normal anatomy to be routinely identified for rectal/anal cancer
  - Small bowel
  - Bladder
  - Femoral heads: to be contoured inferiorly to the level of ischial tuberosity
  - External genitalia
  - Consider remaining large bowel
  - Consider iliac crest when using intensity-modulated radiation therapy

Treatment Planning

Therapy

- Two-dimensional, anatomy-based planning has been the historic standard, from which the majority of data on treatment results and toxicity outcomes have conventionally been derived. Elective nodal irradiation of nonclinically involved regional lymphatics was standard in this approach.
- 3DCRT contemporary treatment paradigms for GI malignancies use planning based on CT-derived targets, for which combinations of coplanar 3D conformal fields are used for EBRT delivery.
- IMRT: IMRT is increasingly used in RT treatment of the GI tract but remains investigational. Its main advantage lies in potential reduction in normal tissue toxicity.

Critical Structures

- Spinal cord: maximum dose, less than 50 Gy.
- Liver: two thirds of the organ, less than 30 Gy; mean dose, less than 25 Gy.
- Kidneys: a renal perfusion scintiscan may be obtained prior to treatment to assess kidney function.
  - The equivalent of 1 whole kidney should be limited to less than 20 Gy.
  - The mean dose for the total kidneys is less than 16 Gy.
  - If the patient has only 1 functioning kidney, exclude two thirds of that kidney from the radiation field.
- Small bowel: maximum point dose, less than 54 Gy; 1 cc, less than 50 Gy; 20 cc, less than 45 Gy. Relative volume limits: up to 10% may receive 54 Gy; up to 15%, 50 Gy.
- Stomach: maximum dose, 54 Gy. Relative volume limits: up to 10% may receive 54 Gy; up to 15%, 50 Gy.
- Femoral head: maximum dose, 50 Gy.

Technical Factors

- 6 to 18 MV photon beam energies; higher energy photons are often required for patients with greater separation.
- Beam shaping with multileaf collimators or individually shaped (5 HVL) custom blocks for normal tissue protection outside the target volume.
- Heterogeneity corrections: if using contrast-enhanced CT scans at the time of planning, density overrides or fusion of noncontrasted scans are required when using heterogeneity corrections in planning.
- Avoid planning on CT images with contrast enemas if near tumor because of displacement effects.

PANCREATIC CANCER

Indications

- Postoperative (adjuvant) chemoradiotherapy
- Definitive chemoradiotherapy for unresectable (T4) disease
- Preoperative (neoadjuvant) chemoradiotherapy in selected patients
- Chemoradiotherapy with 5FU

Localization, Immobilization, and Simulation

- Immobilization and patient position
  - Supine.
  - Can consider prone with belly board in patients who will not have AP/PA field contributions.
- Contrast agents and markers
  - Oral contrast to delineate the small bowel.
  - IV contrast to delineate the tumor and LN; specific use of pancreatic contrast timing protocols will improve resolution.

Target Volume Definition

Neoadjuvant
- GTV
  - Primary tumor + clinically positive LN greater than 1 cm short axis diameter
    - Involved volume best defined on contrast-enhanced MRI or pancreatic phase contrast-enhanced CT scan.
- CTV
  - May elect to include immediate primary LN drainage, with a focus only on the highest risk portions of these chains for neoadjuvant therapy.
    - Head lesions: consider celiac, portahepatis, suprapancreatic and pancreatic duodenal LNs.
    - Tail lesions: consider celiac, splenic and lateral suprapancreatic LNs.
- PTV
  - PTV= CTV + 1 cm.

Adjuvant
- GTV
  - None. If STR, then treat remaining GTV per unresectable and include LN below.
- CTV

- Tumor bed plus nodal drainage for initial field with a boost to the tumor bed.
  - Tumor bed defined by fusion of preoperative imaging and surgical clips.
- Pancreatico-jejunostomy and hepatico-jejunostomy (if the entire jejunum is resected, do not include pancreatico-gastrostomy).
  - At-risk LN
    - Head lesions : celiac (proximal 1-1.5 cm of the celiac artery), superior mesenteric (proximal 2.5 cm of the superior mesenteric artery), porta hepatis, suprapancreatic, pancreaticoduodenal, para-aortic (from T11 to L3).
    - Tail lesions: celiac, superior mesenteric, splenic, lateral suprapancreatic.
      - Coverage of the porta hepatis and pancreaticoduodenal lymph nodes should be attempted for body/tail lesions but may be omitted to meet dose constraints on the kidneys.
- PTV
  - PTV = CTV + 1 cm

Unresectable
- GTV
  - Primary tumor + clinically positive LN greater than 1 cm short axis diameter.
    - Involved volume best defined on contrast-enhanced MRI or pancreatic phase contrast-enhanced CT scan.
- CTV
  - Historically, primary draining LN, as listed in the "Adjuvant" section, were included in the CTV; current practice trends are to restrict the size of the CTV to GTV plus 1 cm, then a margin for PTV margin, given limited ability to control primary disease.
- PTV
  - PTV = CTV 1 cm

Treatment Planning
- 4-field technique
  - Initial AP/PA fields:
    - Superior border: T10/T11 vertebral body interspace.
    - Inferior border: L3/L4 vertebral body interspace.
    - Lateral borders: 2 to 3 cm on preoperative primary tumor extent or gross tumor, no less than 2 cm from the vertebral bodies.
  - Initial lateral fields
    - Superior/inferior borders: same as AP/PA fields.

- Anterior border: 1.5 to 2 cm anterior to anterior aspect of preoperative primary tumor or gross tumor and at least 3.5 to 4 cm anterior to the anterior edges of the vertebral bodies.
- Posterior border: split the vertebral bodies in half.
■ Boost field: 1.5 to 2 cm margin on gross tumor or preoperative primary tumor extent.
- Beam arrangement: while AP/PA and 3-field plans incorporating AP/PA and laterals +/- wedges are most common, oblique fields (particularly moving the lateral beams toward anterior obliques) may reduce kidney doses, and noncoplanar beam arrangements may reduce small bowel doses (Figures 7.1 and 7.2).

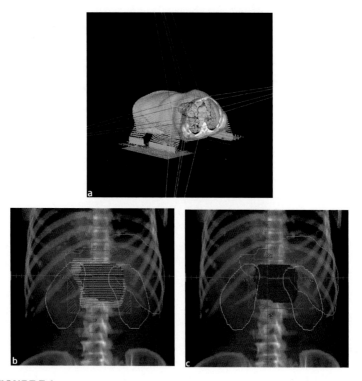

FIGURE 7.1 A 72-year-old woman with borderline resectable pancreatic adenocarcinoma involving the portal vein was treated with neoadjuvant chemoradiation. EBRT technique: 4-field noncoplanar beam arrangement optimized liver sparing (a). The initial fields (b) covered the primary tumor (red) and immediate primary LN drainage (green) with 1-cm radial and 1.5-cm superior/inferior block margins. The cone down (c) covered the primary tumor with 1-cm block margins.

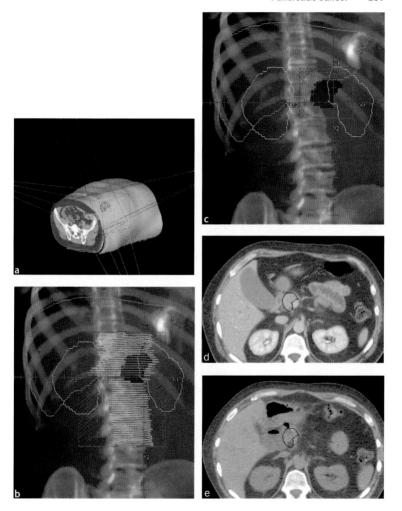

FIGURE 7.2 A 51-year-old man, post-Whipple procedure for adenocarcinoma of the pancreatic head. RT plan: 4-field noncoplanar beam arrangement optimized liver sparing (a). The initial fields (b) covered the tumor bed (red) and associated LN (green). The cone down (c) covered the tumor bed with a 2-cm block margin. The tumor bed was delineated by fusion of the preoperative CT scan (d) to the planning CT scan (e).

Volumetric Planning Goals

- 95% of the PTV should receive at least 95% of the prescription dose.
- No portion of the PTV should receive less than 90% of the prescription dose.
- 99% of the CTV should receive at least 95% of the prescription dose.
- 0.1 cc of tissue is limited to 115% of the prescription dose.
- 1.0 cc of tissue (or 5% of PTV) is limited to 110% of the prescription dose.
- 5 cc of tissue (or 10% of PTV) is ideally limited to 105% of the prescription dose.

Dose/Fractionation

- Conventional fractionation: 1.8 Gy/fx
- Neoadjuvant RT: 45 Gy to CTV, boost GTV to 50.4 to 54 Gy
- Adjuvant RT: 45 Gy to CTV, boost tumor bed and pathologically involved LN regions to 50.4 Gy
- Definitive RT: 50.4 to 54 Gy to GTV

GASTRIC CANCER

Indications

- Postoperative chemoradiotherapy is the most typical indication, with rare selected cases of preoperative chemoradiotherapy or definitive chemoradiotherapy for unresectable disease.

Localization, Immobilization, and Simulation

- Immobilization and patient position
  - Supine with arms above the head.
- Contrast agents and markers
  - Oral contrast to delineate the small bowel.
  - IV contrast to delineate the tumor and LN.

Target Volume Definition

Adjuvant
- GTV
  - If STR, then treat remaining GTV per unresectable and include LN as below.
- CTV
  - Tumor bed

- Coverage of tumor bed elective for resected T1 to T2a lesions with wide margins.
- Include for all stage T2b to T4.
- Defined by fusion of preoperative imaging and surgical clips.
- Preoperative endoscopy reports my help determine surgical bed location.

■ Remaining stomach (include 5 cm of normal esophagus for gastroesophageal junction (GEJ) lesions)
  - If perigastric or other nodal involvement.
  - If surgical margins less than 5 cm.

■ Lymph nodes
  - If nodal involvement or T4 disease, LN at risk defined by the location of the primary tumor.
    - GEJ: perigastric, periesophageal, and celiac.
    - Cardia: perigastric, periesophageal, celiac, splenic, pancreaticoduodenal, and porta hepatis.
    - Body: perigastric, celiac, splenic, suprapancreatic, pancreaticoduodenal, and porta hepatis.
    - Antrum/pylorus: perigastric, celiac, suprapancreatic, pancreaticoduodenal, and porta hepatis.

Unresectable
■ GTV
  ■ Primary tumor + clinically positive LN seen on planning CT (>1 cm short axis diameter).
    - Endoscopy reports may help determine tumor location.
    - IV contrast will aide in the definition of nodal volumes.
    - Oral contrast (5 minutes prior to simulation) aides in the definition of GTV.
    - MRI or PET fusion may aide in volume definition.
■ CTV
  ■ Entire stomach (include 5 cm of normal esophagus for GEJ lesions).
  ■ Lymph node regions depending on location as for adjuvant therapy.
  ■ Recommend treatment with an empty stomach to reduce target volume and CTV variation within set fields. Daily image guidance for confirmation is strongly suggested in this setting.
  ■ PTV = CTV + 1 cm, may be reduced to 0.5 cm with daily image guidance.

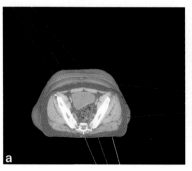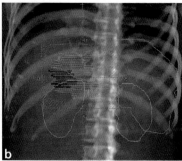

FIGURE 7.3 A 59 year-old man with resected gastric adenocarcinoma, negative margins, 4 involved LN, and soft tissue involvement beyond the serosa. RT plan: 3-field coplanar beam arrangement (a) was chosen to limit dose to the liver and kidney. The initial fields (b) covered the regional lymph nodes (green) and the tumor bed (red).

Treatment Planning

- Conventional 2-field
  - AP/PA arrangement preferred because it provides the best coverage of CTV and respects normal tissue tolerances.
  - Consider lateral field use in patients with anterior gastric location or when AP/PA fields cannot meet normal tissue constraints.
- 3DCRT (Figure 7.3)
  - As needed to achieve normal tissue constraints of kidneys, spinal cord, and liver, particularly when total dose is greater than 45 Gy.

Dose/Fractionation

- For adjuvant therapy, the CTV should receive 45 Gy/1.8 Gy/fx. May consider from 5.4 to 9 Gy boost for positive margins/gross residual disease, as determined by constraints.
- For definitive therapy, the dose to CTV is 45 Gy/1.8 Gy/fx and the GTV total dose is 54 to 59.4 Gy/1.8 Gy/fx.

RECTAL CANCER

Indications

- The once-common postoperative EBRT for resected rectal cancer is being replaced by use of neoadjuvant chemoradiotherapy.
- Concurrent chemoradiotherapy.

Localization, Immobilization, and Simulation

- Immobilization and patient position
  - Prone with arms above the head.
  - Consider belly board to displace small bowel.
  - Simulate and treat with full bladder to displace small bowel.
- Contrast agents and markers
  - Oral contrast to delineate the small bowel.
  - Barium enema to delineate the tumor (caution with respect to tumor displacement).
  - IV contrast to delineate the tumor and LN.
  - Anal marker to delineate the anus.

Target Volume Definition

- GTV
  - Primary tumor + clinically positive nodes greater than 1 cm short axis diameter.
  - PET or MRI fusion typically aides in GTV delineation.
  - Colonoscopy reports may help determine tumor location.
- CTV
  - Lymph nodes for T1 to T3 tumors, include common iliac, internal iliac, and presacral LN as well as the entire mesorectum.
  - Mesorectum
    - Given variations in bladder and rectal filling, expand mesorectal coverage 1 cm anteriorly into the bladder/vagina/prostate.
  - For T4 tumors, also include coverage of external iliac LN.
  - If the anus, skin, or distal one third of the vagina is involved, also include inguinal LN.
- PTV
  - PTV = CTV + 1 cm

Treatment Planning

- Conventional 3-field technique (PA + opposed laterals) (Figure 7.4)
  - Beam weighing typically 2:1:1 for PA and laterals
    - High energy for PA field
    - 6 MV photons for laterals unless wide separation
  - PA field
    - Inferior border: 3 cm below the anal marker
    - Superior border: L5/S1 vertebral body interspace
    - Lateral borders: 1.5 cm on pelvic brim or CTV, whichever is larger
  - Lateral fields

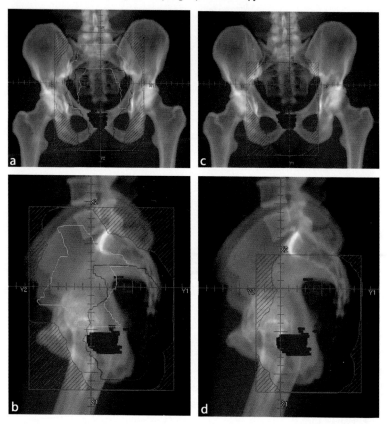

FIGURE 7.4 A 49-year-old man with locally advanced rectal adenocarcinoma, stage T4N1M0, treated preoperatively with chemoradiotherapy. The initial PA (a) and lateral fields (b) covered the primary tumor (red) as well as the internal iliac (green), external iliac (green), presacral (green), and mesorectal (blue) LN. The cone down posterior (c) and lateral fields (d) covered the primary tumor and clinically involved LN (red) with margin.

- Superior/inferior borders: same as PA field
- Anterior border
  - T3 tumors: behind the pubic symphysis
  - T4 tumors: in front of the pubic symphysis to include external iliac LN
- Posterior border: 1 cm behind the sacrum to include presacral lymph nodes
■ Boost field: 2-cm block margin on the GTV
■ Inguinal fields: see "Anal Cancer" section

Volumetric Planning Goals

- 95% of the PTV should receive at least 95% of the prescription dose.
- No portion of the PTV should receive less than 90% of the prescription dose.
- 99% of the CTV should receive at least 95% of the prescription dose.
- 0.1 cc of tissue is limited to 115% of the prescription dose.
- 1.0 cc of tissue (or 5% of the PTV) is limited to 110% of the prescription dose.
- 5 cc of tissue (or 10% of the PTV) is ideally limited to 105% of the prescription dose.
- See "General Principles" section for critical structure dose constraints.

Dose/Fractionation

- Chemoradiotherapy: CTV to 45 Gy/1.8 Gy/fx, boost GTV and presacral LN by additional 5.4 Gy/1.8 Gy/fx

ANAL CANCER

Introduction

- Primary management of anal cancer is definitive chemoradiotherapy.
- Treatment for rare T1N0M0 lesions may include en face electron therapy, interstitial brachytherapy, or contact therapy.
- Surgery is reserved for failure to achieve complete response or for local failures.

Localization, Immobilization, and Simulation

- Immobilization and patient position
  - Supine with arms across the chest or prone in a belly board with arms extended. If using the prone setup for primary fields, may consider supine positioning for the boost (which is typically away from small bowel) so that desquamated patients may be positioned more comfortably.
- Contrast agents and markers
  - Oral contrast to delineate the small bowel.
  - Barium enema to delineate the tumor.
  - IV contrast to delineate the tumor and LN.
  - Anal marker to delineate the anus.
  - Wire to involved inguinal LN.

Target Volume Definitions

- GTV
  - Primary tumor + clinically positive LN seen on planning CT (>1 cm short axis diameter)

- PET or MRI fusion typically aides in GTV delineation.
- Colonoscopy/anoscopy reports may help determine tumor location.
- CTV
  - Lymph nodes at risk include common iliac, external iliac, internal iliac, presacral, mesorectal, perianal, and inguinal.
    - For low-lying anal lesions, inclusion of the superior portion of the mesorectum is controversial.
- PTV
  - PTV = CTV + 1 cm

Treatment Planning

- Conventional 2-field technique (AP/PA) (Figure 7.5)
- Initial field borders
  - Superior border: L5/S1 vertebral body interspace.
  - Inferior border: 3 cm below the anal marker (or 3 cm margin on extent of disease if extending into the anal margin/perianal skin).
  - Lateral border
    - PA: 1.5 cm on pelvic brim.
    - AP: include inguinal nodes with 2 cm lateral to greater sciatic notch
      - Supplement AP photon field with electrons matched to the divergence of the PA field.
      - In vivo dosimetry with TLD can help determine the appropriate electron supplement.
- Cone down no. 1 field borders
  - Lower superior border to the bottom of SI joints.
  - Inferior and lateral borders remain the same.
- Boost field
  - Indicated for T3, T4, N+, or T2 lesions with residual disease after 45 Gy.
  - Use 2-cm margin on GTV via AP/PA, 3-field (opposed laterals and PA – lowest anterior skin dose), or 4-field (AP/PA/laterals) approach.
  - Alternatively, may use en face perineal electron or photon field with the patient in a frog-leg position depending on the depth of the primary tumor.

- Specific clinical scenarios may favor a 4-field technique: this usually requires higher electron supplement to the inguinal nodes, which can result in greater inguinal desquamation.

Volumetric Planning Goals

- 95% of the PTV should receive at least 95% of the prescription dose.
- No portion of the PTV should receive less than 85% of the prescription dose.

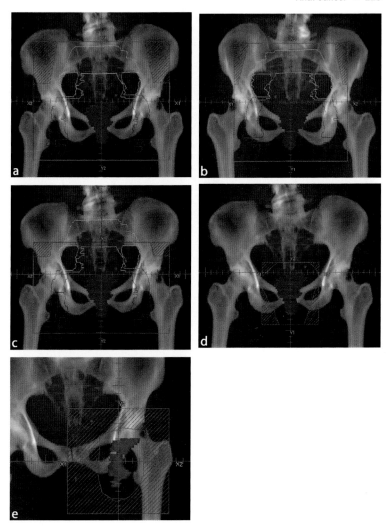

FIGURE 7.5 A 57-year-old woman with locally advanced squamous cell carcinoma of the anus was treated with definitive chemoradiotherapy. Note the medial position of inguinal LN facilitating a 2-field approach. Initial AP (a) and PA (b) fields covered the internal iliac (green), external iliac (green), presacral (green), mesorectal, and inguinal (blue) LN as well as the primary tumor (red). First cone down consisted of similar fields to AP/PA but with the superior border dropped to the bottom of the SI joints; the anterior cone down field is shown (c). The final cone down (d) covered the primary tumor with a 2-cm block margin. Because both inguinal regions were involved, they were boosted an additional 9 Gy with 12 MeV electrons to give a total dose of 54 Gy to the inguinal LN; the left inguinal electron field is shown (e).

- 99% of the CTV should receive at least 95% of the prescription dose.
- 0.1 cc of tissue is limited to 115% of the prescription dose.
- 1.0 cc of tissue (or 5% of the PTV) is limited to 110% of the prescription dose.
- 5 cc of tissue (or 10% of the PTV) is ideally limited to 105% of the prescription dose.
- See "General Principles" section for critical structure dose constraints
  - For external genitalia, attempt to limit
    - 50% to less than 20 Gy
    - 95% to less than 40 Gy
  - For iliac crest, may attempt to limit
    - 50% to less than 30 Gy
    - 95% to less than 50 Gy

Dose/Fractionation

- CTV to 45 Gy/1.8 Gy/fx
  - Field reduction to cone down no. 1 after 30.6 Gy.
- T3, T4, or T2 lesions with residual disease after 45 Gy should receive an additional 9 to 14.4 Gy to the GTV via boost field.
  - T2 dose goal, 45 to 50.4 Gy
  - T3 dose goal, 54 Gy
  - T4 dose goal, 54 to 59.4 Gy
- Clinically negative inguinal LN should receive a minimum of 36 Gy, measuring prescription depth on CT (classically, 3 cm has been used; this may underdose thicker patients).
- Clinically positive inguinal LN should receive a minimum of 45 Gy.
  - Boost additional 5.4 to 9 Gy depending on LN size and clinical response.
- Clinically positive pelvic LN may be boosted along with primary boost field for an additional 5.4 to 9 Gy above 45 Gy CTV dose depending on LN size and clinical response.

8 Genitourinary Radiotherapy

**Mohammad K. Khan, Rahul D. Tendulkar,
Kevin L. Stephans, and Jay P. Ciezki**

GENERAL PRINCIPLES

- Common principles when approaching radiotherapy planning for patients with genitourinary (GU) cancers include simulation techniques, definition of dose-limiting structures, dose constraints, and planning principles.

Localization, Immobilization, and Simulation

- Volumetric treatment planning (CT simulation on a flat surface) for definition of GTV, CTV, and PTV.
- Patient position: supine, with arms folded on the chest.
- Immobilization: use a knee sponge, with the feet banded together in a comfortable and reproducible position. Immobilization using custom molds can be considered.
  - A range of immobilization systems are available and include body molds, vacuum-loc bags, and thermoplastic mesh.

- Contiguous spiral CT slices acquired with 3-mm slice acquisition level.
- At minimum, include the L4-L5 intervertebral disk level to 1 to 2 cm below the lesser trochanteric region of the bilateral femoral heads for most GU sites.
- Contrast agents may be considered:
  - Oral contrast to delineate the bowel.
  - 100 cc bladder contrast mixed with air.
  - 10 cc urethral contrast with penile clamp to delineate the urethra and penile bulb.
  - Rectal contrast.
  - Intravenous contrast to help delineate major blood vessels and nearby lymph nodes.
- MRI in select cases (eg, for better soft tissue definition of prostate apex, penile bulb, bladder primary, and extraprostatic extension).

Image Guidance for Localization and Daily Treatment Verification

- Obese patients and postoperative patients are routinely limited to CBCT, US, or implanted fiducials. Hip prosthesis may limit the use of CBCT owing to artifact.
- No one form of IGRT is superior to another. Selection of image guidance methods depends on patient factors and availability.

Target Volumes and Organs of Interest Definition

- Normal anatomy routinely identified (Table 8.1).
  - Kidneys: contour left and right separately.
  - Bowel: contour individual loops or as a section of bowel beginning at the level of L5-S1 to the rectosigmoid junction. Consider contouring from L3-L4 if concerned about hot spots in bowel higher in the pelvic region.
  - Rectum: begin contouring at the level of rectosigmoid junction inferiorly to the level of the anal verge or at least 15 cm in length measured superiorly from the anal verge.
  - Bladder: contour the bladder from the level of the urachus to the bladder neck at the level of prostate.
  - Prostate: begin contouring at the level of the bladder neck and extend the contour inferiorly to the level of the prostate apex. The prostate apex is located about 1 to 1.5 cm above the urethrogram beak. Alternatively, consider using MRI to define the apex.
  - Penile bulb: located at the level of the beak on a urethrogram.

- Seminal vesicles (as needed): contour the proximal 1 to 2 cm if treating intermediate and high risk prostate cancer. Consider treating the entire seminal vesicles if they are grossly involved.

- Femoral heads: contour the left and right separately beginning at the top of the femoral head within the acetabulum and extend inferiorly to the level of the lesser trochanter bilaterally.

- Lymph nodes (as needed) (Figure 8.1) (1): start contouring at the level of L5/S1 for most GU sites as described.

  - Common iliac: start at level of L5/S1 to the bifurcation at which the common iliacs give rise to the external and internal iliacs.

  - Internal iliacs: contour the internal iliacs inferiorly to the level of the prostate.

  - External iliacs: contour the external iliacs inferiorly to the level of the top of the femoral heads bilaterally at the level of the inguinal ligament.

  - Presacrals: contour between S1 and S3.

  - Obturators: contour between the level of the femoral heads superiorly to the superior most portion of the pubis symphysis inferiorly. Ensure an 18-mm-wide strip extending from the external and internal iliacs.

- Testicles (as needed): right and left separately.

- Penis (as needed): starting at the level of penile bulb and including the corpus spongiosum, corpus cavernosum, the shaft, and the glans penis.

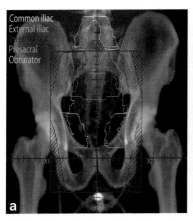 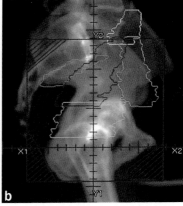

FIGURE 8.1 Example of ports used for a 4-field box technique to treat pelvic lymph nodes. AP projection (a) and right lateral projection (b).

Treatment Planning

Historically, 2-dimensional planning was common. This has been replaced by 3-dimensional conformal or intensity-modulated radiation therapy with increased reliance on daily IGRT. A 2-field (anteroposterior [AP]/posteroanterior [PA]) or a 4-field (AP/PA and laterals) approach for pelvic lymph nodes is followed by boost to primary. Alternatively, IMRT can also be used to treat pelvic lymph nodes to minimize normal tissue toxicity. Quality assurance of IMRT should be accomplished using phantom measurements prior to the start of treatment. Brachytherapy can also be used in particular cases such as that of prostate and select penile and urethral cases.

Lymph Node Irradiation

- Lymph node irradiation for prostate cancer is controversial.
- Routinely used for early stage testicular cancers, bladder cancers, and advanced penile cancers.
- CTV = 7 mm around the lymph node GTV, while excluding the bone, bowel, bladder, and muscle (1).
- PTV = 3 to 5 mm around the CTV.

Technical Factors

Beam energies

- Photon energies 6 to 10 MV are routine; higher energy photons (>10 MV) are not recommended as beam penumbra increases and the beam edge becomes less sharp. In addition, neutron production increases above this energy and can lead to increased scattered dose.

Beam shaping

- Multileaf collimation or individually shaped (5 half value layer) custom blocks for normal tissue protection outside the target volume are routinely used. Clamshell shield is used for testicular cancer in order to minimize radiation to the contralateral testicle.

EXTERNAL BEAM RADIOTHERAPY FOR PROSTATE CANCER

External Beam Radiotherapy Indications

- Intact prostate alone or combined with brachytherapy.
- Postprostatectomy in the adjuvant or salvage setting.

Target Volume Definition for Definitive EBRT: Intact Prostate

- Definition of the GTV.
  - GTV = prostate.
  - Low risk = prostate only.
  - Clinically positive nodes (≥1.5 cm short axis diameter) seen on planning CT or on MRI should be included as part of nodal GTV.
- Definition of the CTV.
  - Intermediate risk = prostate + proximal 1 to 1.5 cm of the bilateral seminal vesicles.
  - High risk = prostate + proximal 1.5 to 2 cm of the bilateral seminal vesicles (consider entire seminal vesicles if grossly involved).
  - CTV = GTV.
- Definition of the PTV.
  PTV depends on the immobilization technique and the particular IGRT technology being used.
  - With Calypso (see below) localization and tracking, 6- to 8-mm margins in all directions, and 4- to 6-mm posterior to the prostate near the prostate/ rectum interface.
  - With CBCT IGRT, 8- to 10-mm all around the prostate and 6- to 8-mm posterior to the prostate near the prostate-rectum interface
  - With US IGRT, larger margins are recommended due to systematic displacement of the prostate due to probe pressure (2): 8- to 12-mm all around the prostate and 6- to 10-mm posterior to the prostate.

Lymph Node Irradiation (LNI)

- Use of LNI is controversial.
- When LNI is indicated, use 2- or 4-field box (Figure 8.1a and b) with field borders as follows:
  - Anterior and posterior field:
    - Superior: L5/S1 or mid-sacroiliac (SI) joint or bottom of SI joint depending on the extent of common iliacs' coverage.
      - Use L5/S1 if there are positive pelvic lymph nodes, may consider a lower border if there are negative pelvic lymph nodes and relatively low risk of lymph node involvement.
    - Inferior: bottom of ischial tuberosity or 1.5 cm below the apex of the urethrogram.
    - Lateral: 1 to 1.5 cm lateral to the pelvic brim.
    - Block regions including the small bowel, femoral head, and unnecessary skin.

- Lateral field borders:
  - Anterior: 1 cm anterior to the pubic symphysis.
  - Posterior: S3/S4.
  - Block regions including the small bowel, femoral head, and unnecessary skin.
- Alternatively, consider IMRT. For lymph node coverage, see section on Target Volumes and Organs of Interest (p. 118). Treatment Planning for IMRT is discussed in the planning section.

Dose/Fractionation

- Intensity-modulated radiation therapy is routine for prostate cancer treatment.
- 72 to 79.2 Gy/1.8 to 2 Gy/fx for low-risk prostate and 75.6 to 79.2 Gy/1.8 to 2 Gy/fx for high-risk prostate.
  - Hypofractionated therapy of 70 Gy/2.5 Gy/fx is reasonable .
- 45 to 50.4 Gy/1.8 Gy/fx to lymph nodes if clinically indicated. Grossly positive nodes can be boosted to a higher dose while respecting normal tissue toxicity.

Image Guidance

- Several IGRT technologies are routinely used and include US, megavolt and kilovolt CBCT, implanted beacon transponder with radiofrequency emission (Calypso), and implanted gold seed fiducial markers.
- IGRT benefits:
  - Reduces systematic errors due to rectal distention and changes in bladder filling.
  - Provides better target localization compared with surface skin marks or bony landmarks.

Planning

Organs containing contrast are manually assigned water density during heterogeneity calculation. Beam arrangements are standardized. A total of 5 beams are used and arranged at 0°, 50°, 100°, 260°, and 310° (ie, ant, RAO, LAO, LPO, and RPO). This arrangement prevents aiming through the rails of the table, which can cause attenuation of the beam on some treatment machines. Lateral fields are avoided if hip prosthesis is noted. Instead, anterior oblique or posterior obliques are used. Use of PA fields are avoided to minimize dose to the rectum. Plan optimization is performed to the PTV via step-and-shoot IMRT. The target is to get 100% of the dose covering 95% or more of the PTV and 99% or more of the CTV. For better homogeneity, 10-MV photons are used. Isodose lines are evaluated for hot spots to ensure that no hot spots are located in or near the rectum. Hot spots elsewhere are maintained below 107% of the prescribed dose.

Critical structures and Suggested Dose Constraints With Conventional Fractionation (Table 8.1)

Normal tissue constraints in the following order for treatment planning: 1= rectum, 2 = bowel, 3 = bladder, 4 = femoral head, and 5 = penile bulb

Of note, IMRT plans may allow for tighter constraints to those listed in Table 8.1.

Dose constraints with standard fractionation are shown in Table 8.1.

Dose constraints with the hypofractionation regimen using 70 Gy/2.5 Gy/fx as follows:

- Rectum:
  - ≤15%, ≥74 Gy.
  - ≤25%, ≥69 Gy.
  - ≤35%, ≥64 Gy.
  - ≤50%, ≥59 Gy.
- Bladder:
  - ≤15%, ≥74 Gy.
  - ≤25%, ≥69 Gy.
  - ≤35%, ≥69 Gy.
  - ≤50%, ≥64 Gy.
- Femoral heads: same as conventional fractionation.
- Penile bulb: mean dose of 51 Gy.

Target Volume Definition for EBRT: Postprostatectomy

- Definition of prostate CTV (Figure 8.2a and 2b).
  - CTV = prostate bed +/- remnant seminal vesicles.
  - Contour the prostate bed beginning at 1.5 cm below the urethrogram beak and continue to the top of the pubic symphysis.
  - Extend the contours laterally to the medial edges of obturator internus muscles bilaterally. Alternatively and more commonly, contour laterally to the SI genitopubic ligament.
  - Anteriorly include the bladder up to the pubic symphysis with gradual reduction posteriorly and superiorly to the bladder for 1–2 cm above the pubic symphysis.

TABLE 8.1 Summary of Contouring Guidelines and Dose Constraints for Intact Prostate

Organ	Contouring Guideline	Dose Constraint	Comments
Rectum	A. Begin contouring superiorly at level of rectosigmoid junction. Continue contouring inferiorly to the level of the anal verge. B. Alternatively start at the anal verge and contour superiorly for a maximal length of 15 cm or until the rectosigmoid junction. in length	1. ≥75 Gy to ≤15% volume 2. **≥70 Gy to ≤25% volume** 3. ≥65 Gy to ≤35% volume 4. ≥50 Gy to ≤50% volume 5. Absolute dose getting above 70 Gy to <10 cm^3	Consider placing metal object at level of anal verge. Post operative dose constraints may be lowered if clinically warranted.
Bladder	Contour bladder from top of bladder at the level of urachus inferiorly to the bladder neck located at the level of the prostate	1. ≥80 Gy to ≤15% volume 2. **≥75 Gy to ≤25% volume** 3. ≥70 Gy to ≤35% volume 4. ≥65 Gy to ≤50% volume	Keep bladder full if treating bladder primary, else partly full if treating other primaries
Bowel	Contour individual loops or as a section of bowel beginning at the level of L5-S1 inferiorly to the rectosigmoid junction	1. ≤50 Gy to ≤66% volume 2. ≤40 Gy to ≤100% volume	
Femoral head	Contour left and right separately beginning at the top of the femoral head within the acetabulum and extending inferiorly to the level to the lesser trochanter bilaterally	≤10% each receive ≥50Gy. **Keep mean dose below 45 Gy.**	
Penile bulb	Located at the level of urethral beak on a urethrogram	Mean dose ≤52.5 Gy	Consider using MRI for better definition

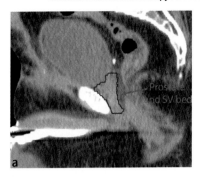

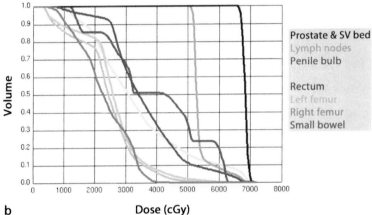

Prostate & SV bed
Lymph nodes
Penile bulb

Rectum
Left femur
Right femur
Small bowel

FIGURE 8.2 Postprostatectomy bed contouring (a) and dose-volume histogram (b).

- Include the area between the bladder and rectum as well as the proximal 2 to 3 cm of the remnant seminal vesicles. Consider including entire seminal vesicles if pathologically involved.
- Consider surgical clips near the prostate bed; however, keep in mind that these are not for RT planning purposes. Do not include hemostasis clips higher in the pelvis if the seminal vesicles are negative for disease.
- Definition of the PTV.
  - PTV = 8 to 15 mm around the CTV.
  - A reduced margin may be used if IGRT and immobilization are used.

Dose/Fractionation

- Typically, 64.8 to 70.2/1.8 to 2 Gy/fx postoperatively.
- A distinction can be made between adjuvant and salvage as follows:

- 60 to 66 Gy/1.8 Gy/fx if adjuvant.
- 70 Gy/2 Gy/fx if salvage.
- 45 to 50.4 Gy/1.8 Gy/fx to pelvic lymph nodes if indicated
- Dose-volume constraints per RTOG 0534 for postprostatectomy radiation as follows:
  - Rectum:
    - ≤25%, ≥65 Gy.
    - ≤45%, ≥40 Gy.
  - Bladder:
    - ≤40%, ≥65 Gy.
    - ≤60%, ≥40 Gy.
  - Femoral heads: same as conventional fractionation.
  - Penile bulb: same as conventional fractionation.

PROSTATE BRACHYTHERAPY

Indications

- Intact prostate, low- or intermediate-risk patients, as a part of or for definitive therapy.

Patient Setup and Preparation (Figure 8.3)

- Preoperatively, patients are instructed to avoid aspirin and anticoagulants for at least 5 days.
- Fleet enema ×2 is given on the morning of the procedure.
- Perioperative intravenous antibiotics (Cefazolin 1 gram × 1 or Ciprofloxacin if PCN allergic) are used.
- Gentamycin 80 milligrams × 1 is added if a patient has a metal implant or a pacemaker.

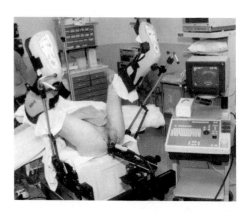

FIGURE 8.3 Patient setup and preparation for prostate brachytherapy.

- General (or spinal) anesthesia is used.
- Patient is placed in an exaggerated dorsal lithotomy position.
- Patient positioning is critical to minimize pubic bone interference during seed placement. Pelvis must be rotated so the pubic arch is elevated.
- The genitalia are taped anteriorly, the perineal skin is shaved, and the rectum is irrigated with a catheter.
- The perineum is prepped with betadine.
- 10 cc of contact jelly is injected into the rectum.
- A US probe is placed within the rectum using a US stabilization device.
- The US stabilization device helps ensure reproducibility from the time of initial US image acquisition and treatment planning to final seed insertion.
- Minimize readjustment of the US stabilization device after a treatment plan has been finalized, as this could lead to a geometrical miss during seed insertion.

Technique (Figure 8.4)

- Radioactive ^{125}I (Iodine-125) (T½ = 60 days, 28 keV photon) or ^{109}Pd (Palladium-109) (T½ = 17 days, 21 keV photon) seeds are commonly used.
- Transrectal US (TRUS) images of the prostate are captured at 5-mm intervals and exported to a treatment planning system.
- Treatment planning can be accomplished preoperatively or intraoperatively.
- Before image acquisition, one should ensure that the prostatic urethra is midline. There should be minimum pubic bone interference using an exaggerated dorsal lithotomy position (Figure 8.3).
- Take measurements of the prostate, including the height, width, length, and volume. These measurements are used for 2 purposes:
  - The number of longitudinal images acquired at 0.5-cm intervals should correspond with the length of the prostate (e.g. a length of 4.5 cm should yield 8-10 axial images for planning, whereas 9 would be an exact match: 4.5 cm/0.5 cm = 9). The subtle differences in the number images planes acquired are due to volume averaging effects.
  - The algorithms used by most commercially available US machines calculate volume using the following equation: ([length × width × height] × 0.52). This approach differs from that used by most treatment planning systems in which the series of volumes of slices 0.5 cm thick are added together. Having 2 independently calculated volumes that agree within 10% of each other adds confidence in the image acquisition and contouring process.
- Commercial planning software is used for contouring the prostate on each slice and for placing seeds within the contoured prostate (Figure 8.4a).
- Stranded or linked sources are placed peripherally. Loose seeds are placed centrally because they are easier to remove as a single source

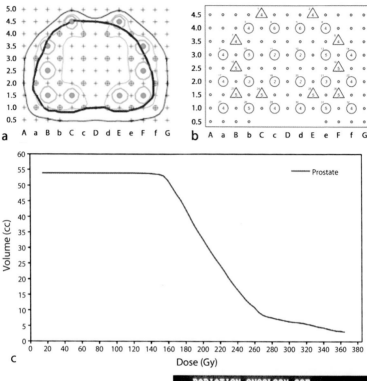

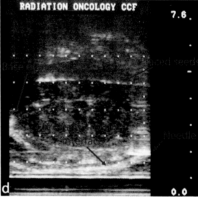

FIGURE 8.4 Isodose distribution (a), number of seeds/needle (b), prostate dose-volume histogram (c), and sagittal ultrasound (d) to guide seed placement.

cystoscopically and spontaneously if misplaced or if placed within the urethra or the bladder.

■ The urethra is readily visualized on the TRUS. Use of a Foley catheter or injected contrast is typically not needed and often obstructs the view of the anterior part of the prostate. Ensure that the urethra is located at the midline of the template (ie, the "D" line in this case) because this helps to minimize the risk of seed placement within the urethra.

■ If urethral visualization is inadequate, consider injecting 3 to 5 ml mixture of lubricant jelly and air or place a Foley catheter +/- contrast. Of note, this may lead to shadowing artifacts anteriorly; thus, this technique should be used sparingly.

■ Image acquisition and physics planning may be done preoperatively or intraoperatively.

■ A final plan will display the number of needles, the number of sources, and the exact geometric location where the needles should be inserted (Figure 8.4b).

■ Preplan goals as follows:
   ■ Volume getting 100% of dose (V100) = 100%.
   ■ Volume getting 150% of dose (V150) $\leq$ 50%.
   ■ Volume getting 200% of dose (V200) $\leq$ 20%.
   ■ Dose to 90% of prostate should be around 115%.
   ■ Central prostatic dose should be <150% of planned dose.

■ A final DVH should be analyzed to ensure that it meets the specified goal (Figure 8.4c).

■ Radioactive seeds are loaded into needles according to the plan.

■ The number of seeds needed is usually around 80 to 100 for ^{125}I but can vary significantly depending on the volume of the gland, the geometry of the implant, the prescription dose, and the source strength per seed.

■ Figure 8.5 shows the total implant activity versus prostate volume. Checking this graph against the case being planned helps reduce prescription errors (e.g. if the total prescription dose was not set properly, one can see this by checking this graph. The plan will not plot in the area of the graph consistent with its volume-activity ratio).

■ The needles are then inserted into the perineum under US guidance.

■ Start placement of needles in the axial coordinate farthest from the TRUS probe to minimize image distortion during seed placement.

■ One should pay close attention to the rectal-prostate interface at the prostate apex during needle placement to minimize risk for seed placement within the rectum (Figure 8.4d).

■ Cystoscopy is indicated if blood is present at the urethral meatus.

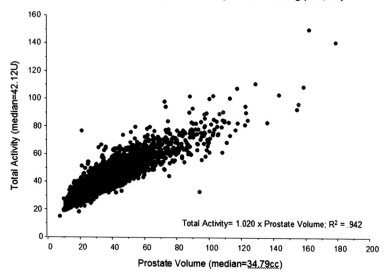

Prostate Volume vs Total Activity for OR Planning (N=2,432)

Total Activity= 1.020 x Prostate Volume; R^2 = .942

FIGURE 8.5 Prostate volume versus total activity.

- Survey meter measured 1 meter from patient must be less than 1 millirem per hour (1 mR/h) for the patient to be discharged for I-125 and Pd-103.
- Survey meter measurements are also taken on contact with patient surface and 10 cm from the patient.

Target Volume Definition for Prostate Brachytherapy

- Definition of prostate GTV:
  - GTV = prostate for low risk.
  - GTV = prostate + 0.5 to 1 cm of the proximal seminal vesicles for intermediate and high risk.
  - Contour the prostate on each slice at 5-mm intervals.
- Definition of the CTV:
  - CTV = GTV.
- Definition of the PTV:
  - PTV = CTV + 5 mm radial margins at the apex and base and 3 to 5 mm elsewhere. Smaller margins of 0–2 mm are used posteriorly near the rectum.
  - Smaller PTV margins can be considered for low-risk patients.

Postimplantation Patient Directions

■ Give antibiotics (Ciprofloxacin 500 milligram [mg] BID by mouth) for 7 to 10 days.

■ Give α-blocker (eg, Tamsulosin 0.4 mg tablets by mouth at bedtime or Terazosin 5 mg by mouth at bedtime) for 2 to 6 months.

■ Pain is usually minimal postoperation; thus, mild analgesics may be considered.

■ Advise that the patient return around 4 weeks postoperation for a CT scan to evaluate the quality of the treatment plan.

■ The goal is to ensure that the V100 of the rectum is less than 1 cc.

Dose/Fractionation

■ Monotherapy prescription dose is 144 to 160 Gy for ^{125}I and 115 to 125 Gy for [103]Pd during implantation.

■ Combined therapy dose with 45 Gy EBRT dose is 108 to 110 Gy for ^{125}I and 90 to 100 Gy for [103]Pd.

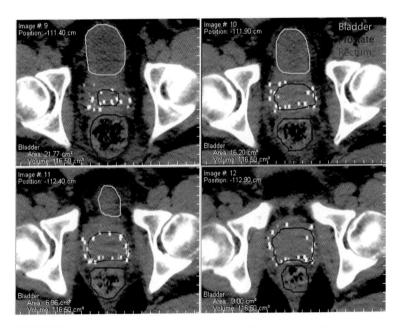

FIGURE 8.6 Postimplantation contouring for quality assurance of prostate brachytherapy.

- The prostate, bladder, and rectum are contoured on each posttreatment CT image slice (Figure 8.6) to generate organ volumes (Figure 8.7a).
- Commercial planning software is then used to determine the location of each seed on the posttreatment CT.
- The location of each seed with respect to the contoured volumes is used to assess the quality of the intraoperative seed placement (Figure 8.7b).
- With monotherapy:
  - Minimum dose to 90% of the prostate PTV (D90) should be between 90% and 130% of the prescribed dose.
  - For ^{125}I, with a prescription dose of 144 Gy, D90 should be higher than 120 to 140 Gy, especially the peripheral zone. This "rule" is not absolute because it does not take into account the fact that cancer is more likely to be present in the peripheral zone of the prostate. If one is faced with a D90 that is less than 120 Gy with ^{125}I the posterior portion of the gland is well above 120 Gy, the implant is likely to be satisfactory without the need to reimplant any cold spots. This algorithm's validity is confirmed by the outcome of patients treated in this manner, where the prostate cancer–specific death rate at 10 years equals that of radical prostatectomy (e.g. 1%).
  - For ^{103}Pd, with prescription dose of 125 Gy, D90 should be higher than 100 Gy.
  - At least 80% of the prostate volume should get at least 100% of the pre-scribed dose (V100 >80%).

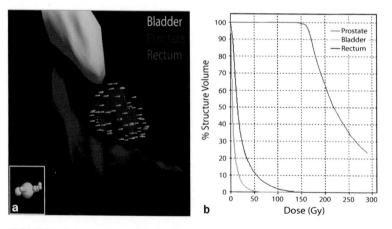

FIGURE 8.7 Postimplantation 3D rendering (a) and dose-volume histogram (b) for quality assurance of prostate brachytherapy.

- Urethral dose should be limited to 150% (216 Gy) of the target dose with ^{125}I.
- Volume of the rectum receiving 100% of the prescribed dose should be less than 1 cc (3-6).

BLADDER CANCER

RT indications

- Bladder preservation: as part of an induction and consolidation approach, usually after transurethral resection of bladder tumor.

Localization, Immobilization, and Simulation

- Pelvic immobilization (eg, vacuum-locking bag is recommended).
- Patient is advised to empty bladder prior to simulation.
- Bladder is filled with contrast (post-void residual volume + 15 cc contrast) and air (15 cc).
- Voided bladder is more reproducible at the time of treatment and minimizes treatment volume when treating the whole bladder.
- Use full bladder volume when boosting as cone down to the tumor to minimize dose to the bowel.
- Air bubble in the bladder marks anterior bladder.
- Rectal contrast is recommended when opposed lateral boost fields are used.
- Bladder fiducials (cystoscopically placed) are optional.
- The bladder wall is 0.5 to 1 cm beyond contrast on radiograph (contrast outlines inner wall of bladder).
- Contiguous spiral CT slices are acquired with 3-mm slice acquisition beginning at the L4-L5 intervertebral disk level down to 1 to 2 cm below the lesser trochanteric region of bilateral femoral heads.

Target Volume Definition

- Definition of the GTV
  - GTV_{tumor} = pre–transurethral resection of bladder tumor (as assessed on cystoscopy, CT, PET, or MRI).
- Definition of the CTV
  - CTV_{pelvis} = $GTV_{bladder}$ + proximal urethra + prostate and prostatic urethra (in men) or proximal 2 cm of the female urethra + regional lymphatics (internal iliac, external iliac, and obturators).
  - $CTV_{bladder}$ = GTV_{tumor} + bladder + bladder wall thickness (0.5-1 cm beyond contrast).

- $CTV_{boost} = GTV_{tumor}$.
- Definition of the PTV (typically included as part of the 4-field approach)
  - $PTV_{pelvis} = CTV_{pelvis} + 2$ cm.
  - $PTV_{bladder} = CTV_{bladder} + 2$-cm margin.
  - $PTV_{boost} = CTV_{tumor} + 2$-cm margin.

Special Considerations

- Preinduction and postinduction cystoscopies are important for bladder and tumor mapping as well as for tumor response assessment.
- The tumor map is used for the boost portion of radiation during the consolidation phase of treatment.

Treatment Planning

- A 4-field approach is routine.
- 4-field approach (Figure 8.8a and b):
  - Use AP, PA fields weighted 70% with borders as follows:
    - Superior: mid-SI joint (or L5/S1).
    - Inferior border: bottom of the obturator foramen (or ischial tuberosities).
    - Lateral border: 1.5 to 2 cm on the bony pelvis, block femoral heads.
  - Use opposed lateral fields weighted 30% with borders as follows:
    - Anterior border: 1- to 3-cm margin on the bladder (seen as air bubble).
    - Posterior border: split the rectum (or 2-3 cm behind the bladder).

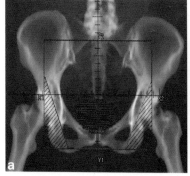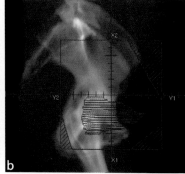

FIGURE 8.8 Four-field box technique for bladder cancer using AP/PA (a) and opposed laterals (b); bladder CTV is delineated in red.

■ Cone down:
  ■ Wait 3 weeks after 39 to 42 Gy/1.8 to 2 Gy/fraction of induction chemo-radiotherapy and repeat cystoscopy. A 3-week wait is not absolute. A shorter wait time can be considered. Do not want in medically inoperable patients.
  ■ Cone down to tumor + 2 cm after complete response for a total dose of 64.8 Gy/1.8 Gy/fraction.

Dose/Fractionation

■ Either BID irradiation regimen or once a day (Qday) regimen can be used.
■ For BID regimen, induction chemotherapy is followed by irradiation as follows:
  ■ First 5 days:
    • CTV_{pelvis}: 1.6 Gy/d × 5 days in the morning.
    • $CTV_{bladder}$: 1.5 Gy/d ×5 days in the evening.
  ■ Next 8 days:
    • CTV_{pelvis}: 1.6 Gy/d ×5 days per week in the morning.
    • CT_{boost}: 1.5 Gy/d × 5 days per week in PM.
  ■ After 40.3 Gy to the tumor, patients undergo repeat cystoscopy followed by consolidation over 8 days as follows:
    • CTV_{pelvis}: 1.5 Gy/d BID for a total pelvis dose of 44.8 Gy.
    • CTV_{boost}: total dose, 64.3 Gy.
  ■ The total dose of 64.3 should be delivered in 42 fractions over 9 weeks.
■ Qday regimen can be used as follows:
  ■ First 10 days:
    • CTV_{pelvis}: 2 Gy/d.
  ■ Next 4 days:
    • $CTV_{bladder}$: 2 Gy/d.
  ■ Next 6 days:
    • CTV_{boost}: 2 Gy/d for a total dose of 40 Gy.
  ■ Patient should undergo repeat cystoscopy followed by consolidation as follows:
    • CTV_{pelvis}: 2 Gy/d ×12 days for a total dose of 64 Gy to CTV_{boost} and 44 Gy to CTV_{pelvis}.
  ■ The total dose of 64 Gy to CTV_{boost} should be delivered in 32 fractions over 10 weeks.
  ■ Alternative Qday regimen may consist of 1.8 Gy/d until the pelvis regimen reaches 39.6 Gy. This is followed by reassessment with a cystoscopy followed by a boost to 64.8 Gy.

Treatment Planning

- In addition to the dose constraints presented in the "General Principles" section, also consider the following:
  - 50% of the rectum should be below 55 Gy.
  - Maximum dose to the femoral heads should be limited to 45 Gy.
  - Maximum dose to the small bowel is less than 50 Gy.
- Three-dimensional conformal planning is used for treatment planning.
- Intensity-modulated radiation therapy is not standard.
- Consider wedges in the lateral fields to compensate for an anterior abdominal slope.
- Multiple field arrangements may be used to optimize treatment, including 4-field, opposed lateral, and 3 to 4 oblique fields; the choice depends on physician experience, tumor location, target volume, and dose from initial large pelvic portals to dose-limiting structures such as femoral heads, rectum, and small intestines.
- Preferential weighting may aid in limiting the rectal and femoral head doses, much of the bladder is anterior, and therefore, weighing to the anterior field may be favorable.
- Weighting the AP/PA 70%, laterals 30% may also help spare femoral heads.
- Saving lateral beams for boost may spare more bladder volume.

TESTICULAR CANCER

Indications

- For early-stage (I-IIB) seminomas, external beam radiation is used in the adjuvant setting.

Target Volume Definition

A "dogleg" or a "hockey-stick" setup is historically the standard for regional CTV nodal coverage.

Treatment limited to the para-aortics can be considered in favorable early-stage seminomas (7).

- Definition of the GTV:
  - Not applicable in the adjuvant setting.
- Definition of the CTV:
  - CTV = para-aortics +/- ipsilateral pelvic lymph nodes. Use a 0.5- to 1-cm margin around the nodes without expanding into the bladder, rectum, muscle, and bone.
  - $CTV_{node} = GTV_{node} + 2$ to 3 cm.

- Definition of the PTV (typically included as part of a 2- or 4-field approach):
  - PTV = CTV + 0.3 to 0.5 cm.
  - $PTV_{node} = CTV_{node}$ + 0.3 to 0.5 cm.
- "Dogleg" field borders (Figure 8.9a):
  - Superior: T10/T11 intervertebral disk.
  - Inferior: mid-obturator foramen.
  - Lateral margins: 2 to 3 cm lateral to the vertebral bodies, including the transverse processes bilaterally.
  - Include the left renal hilum for tumor in the left testicle.
  - Ipsilateral margin: continue to L5/S1 intervertebral body then diagonally to the lateral edge of the acetabulum then vertically down to the mid-obturator level.
  - Contralateral margin: continue to mid L5-S1 then angle diagonally in parallel with the ipsilateral border to the level of the superior most aspect of the acetabulum. Then, the field follows vertically inferior to the median border of the obturator foramen in a fashion parallel to the ipsilateral margin.
    - Para-aortic field borders (Figure 8.9b):
      - Superior: T10/T11 intervertebral disk.
      - Inferior: L5/S1 intervertebral disk.
      - Lateral: 2 to 3 cm lateral to the vertebral disk. Include the left renal hilum if there is tumor in the left testicle. Careful attention should

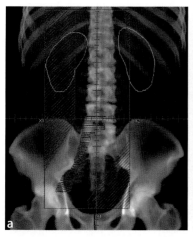
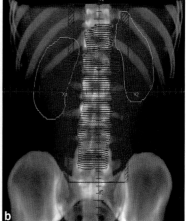

FIGURE 8.9 Dogleg (a) and PA (b) field setup for early stage seminoma. Kidneys outlined in green, CTV in red.

be paid to renal doses because large lateral borders will result in increased dose to the kidney.

Dose/Fractionation

- 25.5 Gy/1.5 to 1.7 Gy/fx, or 20 to 30 Gy in 2 Gy/fx
- Grossly positive lymph nodes greater than 2 cm can be boosted an additional 10 Gy with 2- to 3-cm margins.
- 20 and 30 Gy demonstrated similar efficacy, with reduced adverse effects in a randomized trial for stage I seminoma (8).
- Stage II or recurrent cancer after observation should be treated with a dog-leg setup to ~25 Gy.
    - Boost lymph nodes 2 cm or greater to 30 to 35 Gy.
    - Boost 2- to 5-cm lymph nodes to 35 Gy.

Treatment Planning

- Anteroposterior/posteroanterior setup is most common.
- Planning target volume should be readily covered with the standard AP/PA setup.
- Complex field arrangement such as IMRT or 3-dimensional CRT should be avoided because they may increase the integral dose relative to a simple AP/PA setup.
- Photons 10 to 18 MV allow for greater skin sparing while increasing the homogeneity of dose distribution relative to lower energy photons.
- Clamshell should be used to minimize dose to the contralateral testicle.
- Double thickness midline block can further decrease testicular dose.

PENILE CANCER

Indications

- Brachytherapy or EBRT may be used for early-stage (T1,T2, and select T3) lesions in an attempt for penile preservation.
- Combined modality approach can be considered for more advanced lesions.

Brachytherapy

- Can be considered for lesions less than 4 cm with invasion of corpora cavernosa less than 1 cm.
- Typically reserved for T1, T2, and select T3 lesions.
- Consider limiting brachytherapy for volume size less than 8 cc and use of less than 6 needles to minimize adverse effects.
- Treat full thickness of the penile shaft because clinical staging maybe unreliable because it may underestimate the extent of the disease.

- LDR or HDR can be used.
- Place interstitial templates on each side of the penile shaft for stabilization and insertion of the needles.
- Enclose the penile shaft in a supportive styrofoam collar.
- Needles are inserted perpendicular and parallel, 1 cm apart, and typically in 3 planes with 2 to 3 needles in each plane for larger lesions.
- Often, needles are inserted as a single plane of 2 to 3 needles for smaller lesions.
- Target volume is tumor plus 1.5 to 2 cm.
- Dose is 60 to 65 Gy (46-50 Gy at the center of the organ and limit urethra dose to 50 Gy).
- Radiation is delivered over 6 to 7 days.

External Beam RT

- A patient ineligible for brachytherapy based on tumor size (>4 cm), depth of invasion (>1 cm), and stage (T2 lesions >4 cm, most T3) can be considered for EBRT.

Simulation/immobilization

- Simulate the patient with immobilization using a bolus wax.
- Techniques to immobilize the penile shaft include wax mold, Presplex block, plastic cylinder, and water bath.
- The purpose of immobilization technique is to provide dose buildup to the surface of the shaft and for reproducibility of the geometry during a course of fractionated radiotherapy.
- Treat in frog-leg position if there are plans to treat the inguinal region (eg, in cases when nodes are positive or unknown).

Target definition

- Pelvic nodal irradiation can be omitted if deep pelvic lymph nodes are clinically negative.
- Treat only the involved groin if the contralateral side has been surgically staged and found to be negative, including the deep pelvic nodes.

Dose/technique

- Use parallel-opposed photon beams to 45 to 50.4 Gy to the whole penile shaft using opposed laterals followed by a cone down to 60 to 70 Gy to 2-cm margin.
- For in situ tumor (T_{is}), consider 125 to 250 kV orthovoltage or 13 MeV electrons to 35 Gy in 10 fx of 3-5 Gy/fx.
- Use AP/PA to cover inguinal LN. Negative nodes should receive 50 Gy. Palpable/unresectable nodes should be treated to 70 to 75 Gy.
- Refer to the "Anal Cancer" section on radiation to the inguinal region.

URETHRAL CANCER

- Management of urethral cancer with radiotherapy depends on tumor location, extent of disease, patient status, and patient sex because surgery is the primary management tool.

Male Urethra

- Bulbomembranous urethral tumors can be treated with AP/PA fields to 45 Gy/1.8 Gy/fx followed by a perineal and inguinal to 70 Gy if positive.
- Lesions of the prostatic urethra are treated similar to prostate cancer.
- Radiation for distal urethral cancers is similar to radiotherapy for penile cancers (see "Penile Cancer" section).
  - Interstitial brachytherapy can be considered for low-grade distal lesions measuring less than 4 cm in size at stage T1 or early T2.
    - The Memorial hospital or Syed template can be used with a 3-way Foley catheter for urine drainage, stabilization of the implant, and irrigation of the bladder if needed.
    - Six needles are placed 1 cm in apart around a 1-cm radius about the urethra.
    - Volume of implant is tumor + 1- to 2-cm margin.
    - Dose is 60 Gy with brachytherapy alone or 20 to 30 Gy combined with an EBRT dose of 45 Gy to a total dose of 65 to 75 Gy.

Female Urethra

- Early-stage lesions of the anterior distal one-third urethra:
  - May be treated with radiation therapy alone with interstitial or a combination of interstitial and EBRT.
  - Inguinal lymph nodes should be treated for more invasive disease and if clinically node positive.
- Urethral meatus carcinomas can be treated with interstitial ^{192}Ir LDR implant consisting of 8 to 12 needles arranged in an arc around the urethral orifice to a dose of 60 to 70 Gy at 0.4 Gy/h. Treatment volume is typically tumor + 1 to 2 cm.
- Posterior urethral lesions or lesions involving the entire length of the urethra have potential for bladder involvement. Thus, they should be considered for preoperative radiotherapy followed by exenterative surgery (transpubic approach is common) with inguinal lymph node dissection and urinary diversion.
- For larger tumors with extension into the labia, vagina, entire urethra, or base of the bladder:
  - Consider combined EBRT + brachytherapy implant.

- External beam should include the pelvic and inguinal lymph nodes in a manner analogous to anal cancer to a treatment dose of 45 Gy to the whole pelvis, followed by a boost of 10 to 15 Gy to positive nodes via reduced fields. The perineum should be flashed to cover the entire urethra.
- The primary site is boosted using brachytherapy via a vaginal cylinder to a dose of 60 Gy to the entire urethra.
- An interstitial implant can then be used to further boost the tumor dose to a total dose of 70 to 80 Gy.

REFERENCES

1. Lawton CA, Michalski J, El-Naqa I, et al. RTOG GU radiation oncology specialists reach consensus on pelvic lymph node volumes for high-risk prostate cancer. *Int J Radiat Oncol Biol Phys.* 2009;74:383–387.

2. McGahan JP, Ryu J, Fogata M. Ultrasound probe pressure as a source of error in prostate localization for external beam radiotherapy. *Int J Radiat Oncol Biol Phys.* 2004;60:788–793.

3. Mueller A, Wallner K, Merrick G, et al. Perirectal seeds as a risk factor for prostate brachytherapy-related rectal bleeding. *Int J Radiat Oncol Biol Phys.* 2004;59:1047–1052.

4. Waterman FM, Dicker AP. Probability of late rectal morbidity in 125I prostate brachytherapy. *Int J Radiat Oncol Biol Phys.* 2003;55:342–353.

5. Tran A, Wallner K, Merrick G, et al. Rectal fistulas after prostate brachytherapy. *Int J Radiat Oncol Biol Phys.* 2005;63:150–154.

6. Snyder KM, Stock RG, Hong SM, Lo YC, Stone NN. Defining the risk of developing grade 2 proctitis following 125I prostate brachytherapy using a rectal dose-volume histogram analysis. *Int J Radiat Oncol Biol Phys.* 2001;50:335–341.

7. Fossa SD, Horwich A, Russell JM, et al. Optimal planning target volume for stage I testicular seminoma: a Medical Research Council randomized trial. Medical Research Council Testicular Tumor Working Group. *J Clin Oncol.* 1999;17:1146.

8. Jones WG, Fossa SD, Mead GM, et al. Randomized trial of 30 versus 20 Gy in the adjuvant treatment of stage I testicular seminoma: a report on Medical Research Council Trial TE18, European Organisation for the Research and Treatment of Cancer Trial 30942 (ISRCTN18525328). *J Clin Oncol.* 2005;23:1200–1208.

9 Gynecologic Radiotherapy

Susan Guo and Justin J. Juliano

GENERAL PRINCIPLES

- Gynecologic malignancies routinely managed by radiation oncologists include endometrial, cervical, vaginal, and vulvar primary sites.
- Specific dose prescription will be determined by tumor types and treatment approaches, e.g., preoperative, definitive, postoperative, or palliative therapy.

Localization, Immobilization, and Simulation

- Volumetric treatment planning (CT simulation on a flat surface) for definition of GTV, CTV, and PTV.
- Patient position: supine or prone depending on habitus and patient tolerance:
  - Supine position may be more reproducible.
  - Prone position with belly board may be used to displace the bowel anteriorly and superiorly.
- Immobilization with customized body mold that fixes the position of the upper body, trunk, and proximal legs.
- Consider using vaginal, anal, cervical markers to delineate normal structures.

- Contiguous spiral CT slices acquired with 3-mm slice acquisition to cover the entire pelvis.
- IV, PO, or rectal contrast may be used.
- The patient should have a full bladder during simulation and during daily radiation treatments.
- Two separate treatment planning CT scans with full and empty bladder should be fused before outlining the target volumes.

Target Volumes and Organs of Interest Definition for Whole Pelvic Radiation

- Two-dimensional (2D) planning is based on bony anatomy.
- Conventional whole pelvic radiation (WPRT) borders include (Figure 9.1)
  - Superior: L4-L5 or L5-S1 interspace.
  - Inferior: bottom of the obturator foramina to cover proximal two thirds of the vagina or lowest extent of disease with a 3-cm margin.
  - Lateral: 2 cm beyond lateral margins of the true bony pelvis.
  - Anterior: anterior margin of the pubic symphysis.
  - Posterior: through the S2-S3 interface, may extend if necessary for adequate margin.
- When extended field radiation therapy is indicated, the border should be extended superiorly to include T12-L1 interspace.

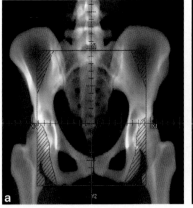 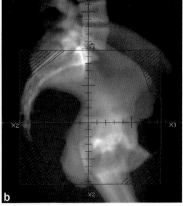

FIGURE 9.1 Conventional borders for whole pelvic radiation: (a) AP view and (b) lateral view.

- CT scan is used to delineate the regions of interest for 3D treatment planning.
- Lymph node group contours for WPRT include the following, using the vasculature as a surrogate (per RTOG 0418 protocol):
  - Lower common iliac nodes: superior limit of the contoured common iliac will be at the top of L5 vertebral body—the PTV should be at the top of L5; therefore, the CTV should be contoured up to 7 mm from the top of L5.
  - Internal iliac nodes (obturator and hypogastric).
  - External iliac nodes up to the level of the top of the femoral heads.
  - PTV of 7-mm margin around the CTV.
  - Include para-aortic nodes if involved.
- Bladder: whole bladder.
- Rectum: volume to include portion inferior to the PTV and superior to level that it leaves the posterior pelvis around the region of the rectosigmoid.
- Small bowel: volume to include at least 2 cm above the PTV and the surrounding loops of small bowel out to edge of peritoneum.
- Femoral heads.
- Sacrum.
- ITV generated from CTV(s) outlined on the full-bladder scan and modified to include the excursion on the empty bladder scan.

Treatment Planning

- 2 (AP-PA) or 4 (AP, PA, right lateral, and left lateral) photon fields.
- IMRT: investigational in the definitive setting, may improve normal tissue sparing in the adjuvant setting.
- 10 MV or higher energy photons are generally used.

Critical Structures

- For extended field radiation therapy:
  - Two thirds of each kidney should not receive more than 18 Gy.
  - Dose to volume of at least 0.03 cc of the spinal cord should be limited to 45 Gy.
- Suggested dose constraints for IMRT per RTOG 0418 (Table 9.1).

Brachytherapy

- A variety of applicators are used, including vaginal cylinder, double tandem, tandem, and ovoids/ring.

TABLE 9.1 Suggested Dose Constraints for Intensity-Modulated Radiation Therapy per RTOG 0418

	% Volume	Gy Constraint
Small bowel	<30	≥40
Rectum	<60	≥30
Bladder	<35	≥45
Femoral head	≤15	≥30

- Common techniques:
  - HDR intracavitary implant: vaginal cylinder:
    - Dorsal lithotomy position.
    - Bladder catheter with balloon is placed.
    - Largest diameter cylinder that can be used is chosen (2.0-3.5 cm).
    - CT simulation in treatment position may be used for volumetric planning.
  - HDR intracavitary implant: tandem and ovoids/ring:
    - Dorsal lithotomy position under sedation.
    - Radio-opaque markers are placed at the anterior and posterior lips of the cervix.
    - Bladder and rectal catheters are placed.
    - Tandem is placed at midline; colpostats/ring is symmetrically positioned against the cervix. The vagina is packed to displace the bladder and rectum; alternatively, rectal blade can be placed.
    - Orthogonal radiographs or CT imaging to assess applicator placement.
  - HDR interstitial implant: Syed:
    - Dorsal lithotomy under general anesthesia.
    - Radio-opaque markers are placed on visible lesions of interest.
    - Obturator placed in the vaginal vault; template introduced over obturator and flush with perineum.
    - Flexiguide catheters placed into template to adequately cover tumor volume.
      - May be done under fluoroscopic or laparascopic guidance.
    - Template is sutured into place at 4 corners.
    - Patients are admitted to the hospital and the template remains in place for 2 to 3 days.
  - LDR implant may also be used for intracavitary or interstitial approaches.

ENDOMETRIAL CANCER

Indications

- Adjuvant radiation therapy for resected endometrial cancer.
- Preoperative radiation therapy: for stage IIIB tumors precluding upfront radical hysterectomy.
- Definitive radiation therapy: for medically inoperable patients or those with unresectable disease.

External Beam RT in the Adjuvant Setting

- Localization, immobilization, and simulation:
  - Per "General Principles."
- Target volumes and organs of interest definition:
  - 3D planning recommended for full nodal coverage
  - Per "General Principles."
  - GTV: none.
  - CTV: lymph node delineation per general principles:
    - Include presacral nodes if cervical stromal invasion.
    - Include entire length of the vagina for patients with stage IIIB disease.
    - Include para-aortic nodes if involved.
  - PTV: per "General Principles."
- Treatment Planning.
  - Per general principles.
- Dose:
  - For WPRT alone, use 45 to 50 Gy/1.8 to 2 Gy/fx.
  - If brachytherapy is planned, treat with WPRT to 45 Gy.
  - Deliver 45 Gy to PA LNs if extended field is used.

Brachytherapy in the Adjuvant Setting

- General principles:
  - Given 4 to 6 weeks postoperatively or 1 week after completion of EBRT.
  - HDR brachytherapy delivered with vaginal cylinder (alternatively, colpostats may be used).
- Localization, immobilization, and simulation:
  - HDR intracavitary implant: vaginal cylinder per "General Principles."
- Target volumes and organs of interest definition:
  - Treat the proximal 3 to 5 cm of the vagina.

- Consider treating the entire length of the vagina for clear cell and serous histologies, or stage IIIB disease.
- Contour the bladder and rectum few slices superior and inferior to the active length of the cylinder.
- Treatment planning:
  - Dose can be prescribed to the surface or at depth (typically 0.5 cm from the surface).
- Dose:
  - HDR and post-EBRT: 6 Gy × 2 (at surface) may be used 3 or more days apart.
  - HDR alone: 10.5 Gy × 3 (at surface) weekly. Alternative: 7 Gy × 3 (at 0.5 cm depth) weekly.

Definitive RT

- General principles:
  - EBRT to whole pelvis, as per "General Principles."
  - Brachytherapy can be used alone with small tumor (eg, <2 cm) and no demonstrable evidence of myometrial invasion (Figure 9.2).
- Localization, immobilization, and simulation:
  - MRI should be used to evaluate the depth of tumor invasion, location, and size.
  - Variety of applicators may be used, including double tandem, tandem plus cylinders, or Heyman capsules.
    - Dorsal lithotomy position.
    - Bladder catheter with balloon is placed.

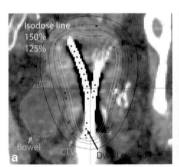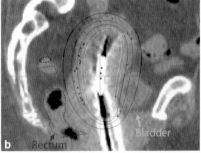

FIGURE 9.2 A 81-year-old medically inoperable woman with endometrial intraepithelial carcinoma treated with HDR brachytherapy with double tandem implant, 7.5 Gy × 5 fx. Brachytherapy plan for definitive treatment of endometrial cancer, coronal (a) and sagittal (b) views.

- CT simulation in treatment position may be used for volumetric planning.
- Target volumes and organs of interest definition:
  - For 3D planning, the GTV and CTV are the uterus.
  - Include the sigmoid colon, rectum, and bladder.
- Treatment planning:
  - For 2D planning, specify dose at 2 cm caudally from the fundus (at midline) and 2 cm laterally.
  - For 3D planning (recommended), contour and prescribe to the volume of the uterus.
- Dose:
  - HDR alone: 7 to 7.5 Gy × 5.
  - HDR and post-EBRT: 7 Gy × 3 after EBRT with at least 72 hours between fractions.
  - There is no current standard dose or fractionation scheme; additional regimens can be found per American Brachytherapy Society guidelines (1).

CERVICAL CANCER

Indications

- Definitive: EBRT with brachytherapy.
- Postoperative: EBRT +/- brachytherapy.

External Beam Radiation in the Adjuvant or Definitive Setting

- Localization, immobilization, and simulation.
  - Refer to the "General Principles" section for full details of WPRT.
- Target volumes and organs of interest definition:
  - 3D planning recommended for full nodal coverage
  - Refer to "General Principles" for normal structures.
  - Delineate the GTV (if applicable) and CTV, including the cervix and full extent of tumor, uterus, paracervical, parametrial, and uterosacral ligaments as well as regional nodes.
    - If the distal third of the vagina is involved, inguinal nodes must be covered, with inferior border as the vaginal introitus.
    - If the posterior vaginal wall is involved, cover the perirectal lymph nodes.
    - If the common iliac nodes are positive, raise superior border for 4-cm margin on known nodes.
  - PTV: per "General Principles."

- Treatment planning:
  - Conventional techniques: either 2 (AP-PA) or 4 (AP, PA, right lateral, and left lateral) photon fields.
  - 4-field pelvis borders: will include GTV and CTV as defined by planning CT.
    - AP/PA: superiorly cover L4-L5, 4-cm margin inferiorly/bottom of the obturator foramen to include the pelvic floor, 2 cm lateral to the bony pelvis.
    - Lateral: per "General Principles"; ensure posterior coverage of at least 1.5 cm behind anterior surface of sacrum.
    - For extended field, include 2-cm margin around uninvolved nodes.
  - Special considerations:
    - AP/PA fields should be used for thin patients or for uterosacral ligament involvement. Consider midline block to avoid excess dose adjacent to the implant and to deliver a higher dose to potential tumor-bearing regions outside the implant, placed at 40 Gy.
    - For stage IIB or IIIB or lymph node–positive disease, may boost parametria an additional 5.4-9 Gy depending on response.
- Dose
  - WPRT: 45 to 50 Gy/1.8 to 2 Gy/fx.

Brachytherapy—Definitive

- General principles
  - Brachytherapy alone can be given for stage IA1 cervical cancer.
  - LDR or HDR can be used with comparable outcomes.
    - Advantages of HDR: no anesthesia, outpatient procedure, inverse treatment planning can be used to optimize source dwell positions and dwell times.
    - Disadvantages of HDR: larger fractions compared with LDR, so implant geometry must be optimal.
  - HDR with EBRT:
    - Generally begins during EBRT week 4, provided appropriate tumor reduction.
    - At least 1 insertion per week is performed, with no EBRT or chemotherapy administered on the day of insertion.
    - If majority of EBRT has been given, then 2 insertions per week are performed (separated by 72 hours) to complete all therapy with an overall treatment time of less than 8 weeks.
    - Applicators include tandem and ring, tandem and ovoids, or tandem and split ring.
- Localization, immobilization, and simulation

- Intracavitary HDR implant: tandem and ovoids/ring per "General Principles."
- Target volumes and organs of interest definition
  - Point A: in the plane of the tandem, 2 cm superior and 2 cm lateral to the external os, where the uterine artery and ureter cross.
  - Point B: 5 cm lateral to the midline at the level of point A, representing the obturator LN.
  - Bladder and rectal reference points defined per "Physics" section.
  - If 3D planning is used, define GTV, high-risk CTV, CTV, and contour normal tissues including the bladder, rectum, sigmoid colon, and vagina.
    - Per Groupe Européen de Curiethérapie and European Society for Therapeutic Radiology and Oncology (GEC-ESTRO) working group guidelines, the high-risk CTV includes the whole cervix and presumed extracervical tumor extension at the time of brachytherapy by means of clinical examination and MRI, including pathologic residual tissue(s) defined by palpable induration and/or residual grey zones in the parametria, uterine corpus, vagina, or rectum and bladder on MRI (2).
- Treatment planning
  - Classically, dose has been prescribed to point A.
  - 3D planning and inverse treatment planning, with resultant optimization of dwell positions and times, are increasingly used to improve target coverage while minimizing dose to normal tissues (Figure 9.3).
- Dose
  - Treat point A to 80 to 85 Gy for early stage and 85 to 90 Gy for advanced stage.
  - Pelvic sidewall dose should be 50 to 55 Gy for early and 55 to 65 Gy for advanced stage.

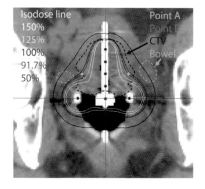

FIGURE 9.3 A 43-year-old woman with adenocarcinoma of the cervix, stage IB2, treated with EBRT 45 Gy with concurrent cisplatin, followed by a brachytherapy boost with a tandem and split ring to total dose of 30 Gy prescribed to point A, at 6 Gy/fx × 5. Brachytherapy plan for cervical cancer: coronal view.

- Limit bladder and rectal doses below 75 and 70 Gy LDR-equivalent doses.
- For HDR, limit bladder and rectal dose to 65% to 70% of the prescription dose.
- Limit upper vagina to 140 Gy and lower vagina to 90 Gy.
  - Dose specification to point A alone is insufficient. The International Commission on Radiation Units & Measurements recommends reporting dose information with technique description, reference volume, dimensions of reference volume, bladder point dose, rectal point dose, pelvic wall point dose, and lymphatic trapezoid dose.
- Special considerations
  - Indications for interstitial implant: bulky cervical cancer (vaginal or parametrial), bulky or vaginal recurrence, and cervical cancer that did not regress during EBRT 3D.

VULVAR CANCER

Indications

- Neoadjuvant chemoradiation for locally advanced lesions.
- Adjuvant RT to the primary site: for positive margins, positive lymph nodes, angiolymphatic invasion, deep invasion.
- Adjuvant RT to lymph nodes at risk: for clinically positive lymph nodes, 2 or more pathologically positive lymph nodes, or extracapsular extension.
- Definitive radiation: for nonsurgical candidates.
- Brachytherapy: as a boost for bulky disease.

External Beam Radiation Therapy

- Localization, immobilization, and simulation:
  - Per "General Principles."
  - Special considerations:
    - Patient position: supine, frog leg position, or legs apart.
    - Wire lymph nodes, vulva, anus, and incision.
  - Bolus groins and vulva as needed.
- Target volumes and organs of interest definition
  - Conventional field borders for 2D planning.
    - Superior: mid-SI joint (pelvic LN–) or L5/S1 (pelvic LN+)
    - Lateral:
      - AP field: include anteroinferior iliac spine (ie, medial two thirds of inguinal ligament), or further if clips suggest more lateral involvement. No need to cover the entire scar if well beyond area at risk.
      - PA field: 2 cm beyond the bony pelvis.

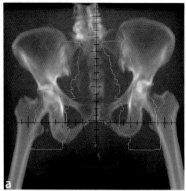

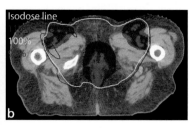

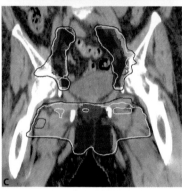

FIGURE 9.4 IMRT plan for a 65-year-old woman with recurrent well-differentiated squamous cell carcinoma of the vulva status post (s/p) multiple resections, presenting with recurrence in left labia and bilateral inguinal lymph nodes. (a) Digitally reconstructed radiograph (DRR) with superimposed nodal (green) and primary (red) CTV; (b) axial and (c) coronal views with CTV delineated in red. Plan consisted of WPRT-45 Gy/1.8 Gy/fx with IMRT, with a concomitant perineal boost of 15 Gy/1.5 Gy/fx twice daily with 18 MEV electrons.

- Inferior: include the vulva, perineal skin, and medial inguinofemoral nodes; generally 2 to 3 cm below the lesser trochanter.
- In select cases, a midline block may be added to reduce dose to distal urethra, vagina, anorectum, and residual vulva.
- ▪ 3D planning is recommended.
- ▪ If treating primary site, contour the vulvar scar with a margin. May be included with pelvic field or en face.
- ▪ If treating nodes, contour unilateral or bilateral groin nodes. Include caudal external iliacs if pelvic nodes are negative, or up to common iliacs if pelvic nodes are positive (Figure 9.4).
- ▪ Treatment planning
  - ▪ 6 MV or higher photons.
  - ▪ Variety of field arrangements can be used.
    - Wide AP field and narrow PA field with partial transmission block placed in the central portion of the AP field.
    - Matched AP/PA fields to include the primary and the pelvic nodes and treat the groins through separate anterior electron fields.

- IMRT increasingly used.
- To supplement vulva for gross disease, use en face field.
- To supplement nodes and respect femoral head tolerance, consider supplemental electrons, half-beam oblique photon fields, or IMRT.

■ Dose:
  - Residual microscopic disease: 45 to 56 Gy/1.8 to 2 Gy/fx for adjuvant therapy.
  - Residual gross disease or definitive therapy: 54 to 64 Gy at standard fractionation (up to 72 Gy without chemotherapy).

VAGINAL CANCER

Indications

■ For stage I patients: consider brachytherapy alone.
■ All other stages require a combination of EBRT and brachytherapy.
■ Radiation therapy is the primary treatment approach for stage II or greater disease.

External Beam Radiation Therapy

■ Localization, immobilization, and simulation
  - Per "General Principles."
  - Special considerations:
    - Tumor and introital markers.
    - Bolus inguinal nodes if needed.
■ Target volumes and organs of interest definition
  - Extend pelvic field border inferiorly to cover the entire vagina and 3 cm below the lowest extent of the disease.
  - If distal one third involvement, lateral borders should include inguinofemoral nodes.
    - Superolateral border: anterior superior iliac spine.
    - Lateral: greater trochanter.
    - Inferior: inguinal crease or 2.5 cm below the ischium.
  - Three-dimensional planning is recommended for full nodal coverage.
  - In select cases, a midline block may be added after 20 Gy to decrease dose to the bladder and rectum when brachytherapy is planned after EBRT.
■ Treatment planning
  - AP-PA or 4-field.
  - 6 MV photons or higher are generally used.

Dose

■ For WPRT alone, 45 to 50 Gy/1.8 to 2 Gy/fx.
■ If brachytherapy is planned, treat WPRT to 45 Gy.

Brachytherapy

- General Principles
  - Use intracavitary HDR general principles for lesions less than 0.5 cm in depth. Please refer to "General Principles" for full details of intracavitary brachytherapy.
  - Use interstitial brachytherapy for lesions more than 0.5 cm in depth.
- Localization, immobilization, and simulation.
  - HDR interstitial implant: see "General Principles" for full details of Syed implant.
- Target volumes:
  - Computed tomography scan is done for treatment planning.
  - For intracavitary brachytherapy, use the largest possible vaginal cylinder to improve the ratio of mucosa to tumor dose.
  - For interstitial implants, the depth of the tumor should be delineated to adequately cover the gross disease.
- Treatment planning
  - 3D planning and inverse treatment planning, with resultant optimization of dwell positions and times, are increasingly used to improve target coverage while minimizing dose to normal tissues.
- Dose/fractionation
  - Cylinder
    - HDR doses of 5 to 7 Gy prescribed to a depth of 0.5 cm into the entire vaginal mucosa are delivered once or twice per week, for total dose of 21 to 25 Gy delivered to the entire vaginal length.
    - An additional 21 to 25 Gy is delivered to the tumor volume using a custom shielded vaginal cylinder, in fractions of 5 to 7 Gy prescribing to a depth of 0.5 cm.
  - Interstitial
    - Total tumor volume doses of 75 to 80 Gy from combined EBRT and brachytherapy implant.

REFERENCES

1. Nag S, Erickson B, Parikh S, et al. The American Brachytherapy Society recommendations for high-dose-rate brachytherapy for carcinoma of the endometrium. *Int J Radiat Oncol Biol Phys.* 2000;48(3):779–790.

2. Haie-Meder C, Potter R, Van Limbergen E, et al. Recommendations from Gynaecological (GYN) GEC-ESTRO Working Group (I): concepts and terms in 3D image based 3D treatment planning in cervix cancer brachytherapy with emphasis on MRI assessment of GTV and CTV. *Radiother Oncol.* 2005;74(3):235–245.

10 Lymphoma and Myeloma Radiotherapy

Lawrence J. Sheplan and Roger M. Macklis

GENERAL PRINCIPLES

- Lymphomas represent a heterogeneous group of disease entities, which make the treatment planning details largely case-specific.
- General principles can guide the clinician in planning EBRT for any given patient. These include simulation techniques, definition of targets and dose-limiting structures, dose constraints, and planning principles.
- Specific dose prescription and target volumes will be determined by the specific disease entity.
- Patients must be examined by the radiation oncologist before chemotherapy to fully quantify the initial extent of the disease.

Localization, Immobilization, and Simulation

- Field design for both Hodgkin and non-Hodgkin lymphoma (HL and NHL, respectively) follows the same general principles and will be described in "Target Volumes and Organs of Interest Definition" section.
- Field boundaries and target delineation are currently areas of ongoing controversy, with the trend in planning favoring decreasing sizes of fields where possible. The 3 main approaches to lymph node coverage are the following:
  - Involved field RT (IFRT) and regional field:
    - Considered by most to be the current standard of care.
    - Treats only portions of the classic fields (see "Target Volumes and Organs of Interest Definition" section), either
      - Involved nodal regions only (IFRT).
      - Involved nodal regions and first echelon uninvolved lymph node basins (regional field).
    - Extranodal sites include entire involved organ.
  - Involved node RT (INRT)
    - Treats only involved nodes as defined from pretreatment FDG-PET scans.
  - Total lymphoid irradiation:
    - Currently rarely used.
    - Includes involved and uninvolved lymph nodes.
    - Treats both supra- and infra-diaphragmatic fields.
    - May be more limited and exclude the pelvic lymph nodes (subtotal lymphoid irradiation).
    - "Classic fields":
      - Mantle: includes all major lymph nodes above the diaphragm.
      - Subdiaphragmatic field:
        - Classic field known as the "inverted Y."
        - Includes retroperitoneal and pelvic LN.

Simulation

- Positioning
  - Supine with the neck extended and arms above the head (draws axillary LN farther from the chest wall, permitting more generous lung shielding).
    - Children: consider arms in the akimbo position.
      - Permits humeral head shielding, minimizing tissue folds in supraclavicular and low neck regions.

Immobilization

- A range of immobilization systems are available to position the arms above the head or akimbo in a reproducible manner.
- Palpable lymph nodes should be wired for visualization.

Target Definition

- All patients must have prechemotherapy and postchemotherapy cervical and thoracic CT scans (axillary lymph node areas must be clearly visible on thoracic CT scans).
- Diagnostic CT scans should be performed in the treatment position, including the prechemotherapy PET-CT, which can help pinpoint previously undetected involved lymph nodes.
  - Computed tomography simulation, in the setting of modern radiation techniques (such as 3D-CRT, IMRT, and IGRT) and immobilization devices, is especially important in the setting of INRT. Defined in "Localization, Immobilization, and Simulation."
- The remission status after chemotherapy should be determined for each initially involved lymph node using CT or PET scans per the criteria detailed in Table 10.1.

Target Volumes and Organs of Interest Definition

- The classic lymphoma fields provide the foundation for understanding how contemporary EBRT fields have evolved.
- Accurate understanding of these fields is required to understand long-term results for disease outcome and toxicity data.
- Mantle field (see Figure 10.1)
  - Superior border includes the inferior portion of the mandible and mastoid tip. Inferior border should be near the insertion of the diaphragm (T10-11).
  - Laterally, the field should include the axilla, extending just beyond the humeral heads (split the humeral head).
  - Lung blocks conform to the mediastinal contour, no more than 0.5-cm margins around the involved LN. Include the pulmonary hilar LN. The superior extent of lung blocks is drawn to expose the infraclavicular region (lymphatic channels here communicate with the axillary and supraclavicular LN regions). Therefore, lung blocks should begin at the third rib and extend down laterally to the sixth rib.
  - Laryngeal block may be placed over the inferior half of thyroid cartilage and cricoid cartilage from the start or at 20 Gy (as long as not blocking

TABLE 10.1 Response Criteria for Lymphoma

	IWC CT Criteria	PET Criteria
CR	Complete disappearance of clinically and/or radiologically detectable disease	–CR by IWC with a completely negative PET –CRu, PR, or SD by IWC with a completely negative PET and a negative BMB if positive prior to therapy –PD by IWC with a completely negative PET and CT abnormalities (new lesion, increasing size of previous lesion), 1.5 cm (1.0 cm in the lungs), and negative BMB if positive prior to therapy
CRu	At least a 75% decrease in tumor size	–CRu by IWC with a completely negative PET but with an indeterminate BMB
PR	At least a 50% decrease in tumor size	–CR, CRu, or PR by IWC with a positive PET at the site of a previously involved node/nodal mass –CR, CRu, PR, or SD by IWC with a positive PET outside the site of a previously involved node/nodal mass –SD by IWC with a positive PET at the site of a previously involved node/nodal mass that regressed to <1.5 cm if previously >1.5 cm, or <1 cm if previously 1.1–1.5 cm
Failure	<50% decrease or any increase in tumor size	–PD by IWC with a positive PET finding corresponding to the CT abnormality (new lesion, increasing size of previous lesion) –PD by IWC with a negative PET and a CT abnormality (new lesion, increasing size of previous lesion) of <1.5 cm (<1.0 cm in the lungs)

Abbreviations: BMB, bone marrow biopsy; CR, complete remission; CRu, unconfirmed complete remission; CT, computed tomography; IWC, International Workshop Criteria; PD, progressive disease; PR, partial response; SD, stable disease.
From Refs. 1 and 2.

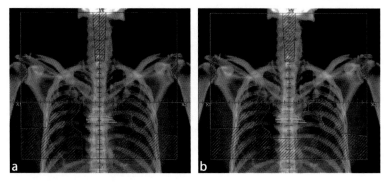

FIGURE 10.1 AP mantle field without (a) and with (b) heart block. Carina is delineated in green for reference.

disease). A posterior cervical cord block (5 HVL) may be considered if the total dose to the cord is calculated to be high (usually for doses >40 Gy, not needed for doses up to 36 Gy).

■ For patients with extension to the pericardium or significant inferior extension of the mediastinal mass, treat the entire cardiac silhouette to 15 Gy, then place a block over the left ventricular apex. A subcarinal block (5 cm below the carina) is placed after 30 Gy to further shield the heart.

■ Inverted-Y field (see Figure 10.2)
  ■ Superior border is matched with the mantle with appropriate gap calculation (overlap at 10-cm depth may be used, gap is on the order of 2–3 cm).
  ■ Right lateral extent to the transverse process or to encompass the involved LN with 1-cm margin and left lateral extent to the rib cage to include the entire spleen (including surgical clips and 2-cm margin to account for respiratory motion).
  ■ Definition of the iliac nodes is best accomplished by lymphangiography or CT, with a 0.5-cm margin around lymphatic bed.
  ■ Inferior border for the para-aortic portion is at L4-L5, after which the pelvic field extends laterally 1.5 to 2 cm past the widest point of the bony pelvis and inferiorly at least to the lesser trochanters.
  ■ Borders may be modified if there is disease that extends past these landmarks or if radiographic studies are used to more accurately delineate nodal anatomy.
  ■ In males, a midline block is placed, and testicular shielding is used to reduce the dose to 0.75 to 3% of the prescription dose, which is predominately from internal scatter.

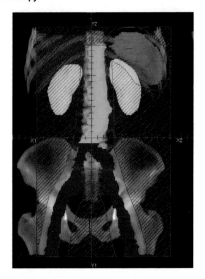

FIGURE 10.2 Inverted-Y field. Para-aortic lymph nodes are delineated in green; pelvic lymph nodes, in red; spleen, in blue; and kidneys, in light blue.

■ In females, the inferior border should not be any lower than the superior level of the sacroiliac joints unless an oophoropexy has been performed, to limit the scatter dose of radiation to the ovaries. A 10-HVL block is placed to shield transposed ovaries after oophoropexy.

■ IFRT: Table 10.2 summarizes the definitions of the major fields (3).

■ INRT: target volume definitions vary according to clinical setting

  ■ Complete remission (CR) or CRu: CTV is the prechemotherapy lymph node volume (excludes blood vessels and normal structures that have been displaced, such as muscle). In case of a CRu, the lymph node remnant should be included in the CTV. A 1-cm margin expansion off the CTV for the PTV is usually considered adequate.

  ■ CR or CRu in the mediastinum: the normal mediastinum is contoured and the CTV should not exceed the lateral mediastinal boundaries except where lymph node remnants are still present in a CRu. The length of the CTV is based on the prechemotherapy volume, but the width of the CTV is the width of the mediastinal mass or lymph node(s) *after* chemotherapy.

  ■ Partial response (PR): GTV is the visible residual disease and should be contoured first. Clinical target volume is the prechemotherapy lymph node volume (excludes blood vessels and normal structures that have been displaced such as muscle). Two PTVs should then be outlined: PTV1 is the expansion on both the CTV and the GTV, usually a 1-cm isotropic margin is considered adequate, and PTV2 is the expansion on the GTV alone, usually a 1-cm isotropic margin is considered adequate.

- If the initially involved lymph nodes are more than 5 cm apart, then separate fields should be devised. If a conventional treatment is used with anterior and posterior fields, the size of the field should be at least 5 × 5 cm.
- Normal anatomy to be routinely identified
  - Lungs (right and left done separately, then combined as a composite lung volume).
  - Heart: from its base (RTOG definition: beginning at the CT slice where the ascending aorta originates and encompassing the great vessels) to the apex.
  - Kidneys: may require blocking to limit dose.
  - Spinal cord: should be contoured on each CT slice.
  - Liver: as needed, based on tumor location and field size.

Treatment Planning

Therapy

- 3D conformal therapy: contemporary treatment paradigms for lymphatic malignancies have been, by and large, based on clinical experience using 2-dimensional treatment planning, and the traditional fields as described in "Target Volumes and Organs of Interest Definition" section were originally meant to be delivered with AP/PA beam arrangements. However, these techniques have been adapted to 3D treatment planning to cover the same areas at risk while restricting the dose to the normal tissues. For the more conformal fields (IFRT and INRT), field arrangements other than AP/PA can be determined by 3D planning to produce an optimal conformal plan in accordance with volume definitions, frequently resulting in much better normal tissue dose profiles. The treatment plan used for each patient is analyzed on the basis of volumetric dose including DVH analyses of the target and critical normal structures.

Critical Structures

- Apart from the kidneys and heart, the doses to the other critical structures are usually well below tolerance for the majority of the dose prescriptions used for the treatment of lymphoma. Lungs, spinal cord, heart, larynx, and kidneys should be blocked as described in "Target Volumes and Organs of Interest Definition" section. Dose limits for all structures at risk as defined elsewhere in this textbook should not be exceeded. Intensity-modulated radiation is necessary on occasion to meet normal tissue constraints (most often for mediastinal disease).
- Kidneys
- Heart

TABLE 10.2 Borders of Involved Fields

Nodal Region	Superior	Inferior
Cervical/SCV (see Figure 10.3)	1–2 cm above the lower tip of the mastoid process and midpoint through the chin	2 cm below the clavicle
Mediastinum/ hilum (see Figure 10.4)	C5-C6 interspace Top of larynx if SCV involved Bottom of larynx if SCV not involved	5 cm below the carina, or 2 cm below prechemotherapy GTV
Axillary (see Figure 10.5)	C5-C6 interspace	Lower tip of the scapula, or 2 cm below lowest axillary node
Para-aortic/spleen (see Figure 10.3, green, area represents PA field)	Top of T11, or at least 2 cm above prechemotherapy GTV	Bottom of L4, or at least 2 cm below pre-chemotherapy GTV
Inguinal/ femoral/ external iliac (see Figure 10.3, red area represents inguinal field)	Mid-SI joint	5 cm below lesser trochanter to include femoral LNs

Abbreviations: GTV, gross tumor volume; ICV, infraclavicular; PA, posteroanterior; SI, sacroiliac; SCV, supraclavicular.

Lateral	Medial	Notes
Include medial 2/3 of the clavicle	SCV uninvolved ipsilateral transverse process, unless involved medial nodes near vertebral body SCV involved Contralateral transverse process	Head hyperextended, arms at the side. Laryngeal block at 19.8 Gy unless there are involved nodes. Posterior cervical cord block if dose >40 Gy. Treat bilateral fields if wbilateral nodes are involved, with posterior mouth block if supine.
Postchemotherapy GTV + 1.5 cm margin	N/A	Include B/L hila + 1 cm if uninvolved and 1.5 cm if involved. Arms up if axillary nodes are involved; otherwise, arms akimbo or at the sides. Treat mantle without axilla if both cervical regions are involved.
Flash axilla	Ipsilateral transverse process. Include vertebral bodies if SCV involved.	Arms up. Includes SCV and ICV nodal regions.
Edge of transverse process, or at least 2 cm from postchemotherapy GTV	N/A	Arms at sides. Include porta hepatis if involved. Contour kidneys for blocks. Consider renal perfusion study.
Greater trochanter, or at least 2 cm from prechemo-therapy GTV. If negative split femur.	Medial border of obturator foramen, or at least 2 cm from prechemotherapy GTV	If common iliac nodes involved, extend to L4-L5 interspace, at least 2 cm above prechemotherapy GTV. Consider slight frog leg. Double shield testicles with clamshell and cerrobend.

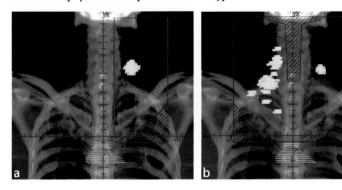

FIGURE 10.3 Cervical lymph node fields: unilateral (a) and bilateral (b). Nodal disease is indicated in yellow, and carina is in green for reference.

Technical Factors

Beam energies
■ Photon energies: 6 to 10 MV.

Beam shaping
■ Multileaf collimation or individually shaped (5 HVL) custom blocks for normal tissue protection outside the target volume are used.

Heterogeneity Corrections

Most dose prescriptions for chest tumors have typically been based on an assumption of homogenous tissue densities. Recently, there has been a move in radiation therapy practice to distinguish the heterogeneous nature to more

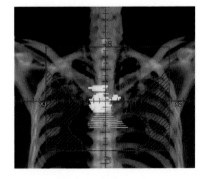

FIGURE 10.4 Mediastinal field. Disease is delineated in yellow, and carina is in green for reference.

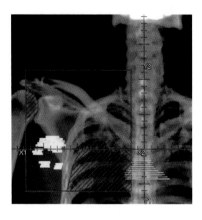

FIGURE 10.5 Axillary field. Disease is delineated in yellow, and carina is in green for reference.

accurately predict dose, dose deposition, normal tissues toxicities, and outcomes. Therefore, heterogeneity corrections are now recommended in general treatment planning.

HODGKIN LYMPHOMA

General Principles

- Stage at presentation determines treatment selection.
- Curative EBRT may be considered for patients with early-stage disease (IA or IIA) as a function of patient and disease variables.
  - Most patients with early-stage disease are now treated with abbreviated chemotherapy and IFRT rather than with radiation therapy alone.
    - Patients with early-stage nodular lymphocyte predominant HL may be treated with radiation therapy alone.
  - Patients of any stage with bulky disease or incomplete response are usually treated with combined chemotherapy and EBRT.

Dose/Fractionation

- There is some controversy with respect to dose in HL.
- Current standard doses range from 30 to 40 Gy with conventional fractionation (1.8–2 Gy/fx), with consideration given to an additional 4- to 10-Gy boost to sites of residual disease or for unfavorable risk groups.
  - Higher doses are favored for larger and less responsive tumors in older patients.
  - Lower doses are favored particularly in pediatric patients and highly responsive lymphomas.

- General dose guidelines
  - Definitive radiation
    - Clinically uninvolved sites, 30 Gy; boost involved sites to 36 to 40 Gy.
  - Adjuvant radiation
    - CR or Cru after chemotherapy: 30 Gy.
    - Pediatric patients: 21 to 24 Gy.
    - With abbreviated chemotherapy for bulky or advanced stage: 36 Gy.
    - Partial response after chemotherapy: 30 to 40 Gy.

NON-HODGKIN LYMPHOMA

General Principles

- Non-Hodgkin lymphoma is composed of more than 40 distinct clinical / histological entities.
- This section focuses on the most common entities: diffuse large B-cell, mantle, follicular, and extranodal marginal zone large B-cell (MALT) lymphomas.

Indolent Lymphomas

Low-grade follicular lymphoma
- One third of cases are early stage, and IFRT is used for cure.

Dose/fractionation
- Doses used ranged from 25 to 40 Gy with conventional fractionation (1.8-2 Gy/fx).

Extranodal Marginal Zone Large B-cell Lymphoma

- Disease of extranodal sites (ie, stomach, salivary glands, Waldeyer ring, thyroid, eye, intestine, etc)
  - Stomach MALTs.
  - RT indicated in the setting of no response or progression after standard management ("triple therapy": proton pump inhibitor (PPI), clarithromycin, and amoxicillin [or metronidazole]).
  - IFRT to stomach, perigastric, and celiac LNs to a dose of ~30 Gy (range, 24-36 Gy).
  - Simulation and planning approach
    - Oral contrast given at simulation.
    - Entire stomach (GTV) and target nodal groups are contoured.

- Stomach contour expanded by several centimeters (~3-5) to encompass target lymph nodes.
- Patient instructed to have empty stomach for simulation and daily for treatment.
- AP/PA fields were traditionally used.
- Complex field arrangements now favored to spare ipsilateral kidney.
■ Nongastric MALTs are usually treated with IFRT to 24 to 36 Gy.
■ Relapsed or refractory low-grade lymphomas.
■ Can be treated palliatively with doses as low as 4 Gy in 2 fx with excellent response and control rates.

Agressive Lymphomas

Diffuse Large B-Cell Lymphoma
Dose/fractionation
■ Treatment is largely determined by stage.
  ■ Early stage: after chemotherapy, IFRT to 30 to 50 Gy (lower doses for better response postchemotherapy and larger amount of chemotherapy cycles, higher doses for the opposite scenarios).
  ■ Advanced stage: may consider RT after chemo for bulky or residual disease, but this is controversial.

Mantle Cell Lymphoma
■ Because this often presents as stage IV, EBRT is indicated only in rare cases, such as combined chemoradiation for stages I-II, especially for bulky disease.

Dose/fractionation
■ Doses range from 15 to 30 Gy.

RADIOIMMUNOTHERAPY

General Principles

■ Two radioimmunopharmaceutical agents are Food and Drug Administration (FDA) approved for the treatment of relapsed or refractory low-grade, follicular, or transformed B-cell NHL, including patients with rituximab refractory follicular NHL; Bexxar is also indicated for transformed CD20+ NHL.
  ■ Zevalin (Spectrum Pharmaceuticals, Irvine, California): ibritumomab tiuxetan, Yttrium-90 labeled IgG κ murine monoclonal anti-CD20 an-

TABLE 10.3 Characteristics of Commonly Used Radioimmunotherapy Agents

Table LJ-Lymph-4	Zevalin	Bexxar
Antibody		
Predose (cold)	Chimeric (rituximab, RTX)	Murine (tostitumomab, TST)
Radiolabeled	Murine IgG1	Murine IgG2
Total dose	250 mg/m^2 × 2	485 mg/m^2 × 2
Isotope	Yttrium-90	Iodine-131
T½ physical	2.7 d	8.0 d
Maximum energy	2.3 MeV β only	0.6 MeV β + 364 keV γ
Mean path length	5.3 mm (~150 cell diam)	0.80 mm
Nontumor uptake	Bone	Thyroid
Dosing		
Platelets >150,000	0.4 mCi/kg	75 cGy whole body dose
Platelets 100-150,000	0.3 mCi/kg (max 32 mCi)	65 cGy whole body dose
Estimated whole body dose	60 cGy	75/65 cGy
Mean tumor dose	1,700 cGy	895 cGy

tibody. A separate isotope, Indium-111, is used for imaging, e-capture decay, 2.8-day half-life.

■ Bexxar (GlaxoSmithKline, Brentford, Middlesex, United Kingdom): tositumomab, Iodine-131 labeled IgG murine anti-CD20 antibody. Dose is based on individual patient pharmacokinetics due to variable excretion.

■ Table 10.3 summarizes the main characteristics of both agents.
■ Contraindications
  ■ Greater than 25% marrow involvement.
  ■ Impaired bone marrow reserve:
    • Prior external beam RT to greater than 25% of the marrow.
    • Platelet count less than 100,000.
    • Neutrophil count less than 1,500.
  ■ Altered bio-distribution based on pretreatment imaging.
  ■ Human antimouse antibodies for Bexxar.

Administration

■ There are several steps to successful radioimmunotherapy requiring multidisciplinary coordination. Table 10.4 summarizes the treatment steps for both Zevalin and Bexxar.

TABLE 10.4 Steps in Administration of Radioimmunotherapy

Day	Description	Details
0	Patient selection	Pretreatment bone marrow biopsy and imaging
0	Cold antibody RTX: Zevalin (Z) TST: Bexxar (B)	Unlabeled antibody (Ab) optimizes the radiolabeled antibody by binding to B lymphocytes and cells with Fc receptors (spleen). Thus, cold Ab blocks binding of the radiolabeled antibody to the normal organs and depletes normal B cells. It also allows deeper penetration and more homogenous distribution. Note: dose for cold Ab in Zevalin administration is 250 mg RTX compared with 375 mg/m^2 for RTX alone.
0 + 4	Tracer dose	A small (5 mCi) dose of radiolabeled antibody is given to assess biodistribution and ensure that pooling does not occur. For Zevalin, Indium-111 is conjugated to ibritumomab instead of Yttrium-90, which cannot be imaged due to its pure β emission. The same antibody/isotope is used for imaging and treatment in the case of Bexxar.
1, 2 (Z) 0, 2, and 6 (B)	Imaging Third Zevalin scan on day 4 is optional.	Gamma camera images are obtained by nuclear medicine. For Zevalin, these scans are used to ensure that pooling does not occur. Bexxar scans are used to calculate the clearance and therapeutic dose because elimination is less predictable than Yttrium-90. This allows for the same area under the curve for patients who have fast and slow clearance. For Zevalin, absorbed dose by the marrow is not predictive of toxicity; hence, detailed dosimetry is not required. Altered biodistribution for Z is defined as high accumulation in the lung > the heart on image 1, or lung > kidney or liver on images 2–3, kidneys > liver on posteroanterior view of day 2 or 3, uptake in normal bowel > liver on days 2 and 3.

TABLE 10.4 Steps in Administration of Radioimmunotherapy (Continued)

Day	Description	Details
7	Thyroid cytoprotection (Bexxar only)	In the case of Bexxar, as the joined antibody is broken down, free Iodine-131 floats in the blood stream, and it can be absorbed by the thyroid, resulting in hypothyroidism. Therefore, 1 day before treatment, Lugol solution/potassium iodide is started and continued for 14 days after treatment to saturate iodine uptake by the thyroid.
8	Treatment	Dosing is based on weight/platelet count for Zevalin and clearance/platelet count for Bexxar (see Table 10.3 above). Infuse over several minutes, monitoring for any infusion related reactions. Radiation safety precautions need to be observed closely.
8	Release instructions	Most (and essentially all Zevalin) patients qualify for immediate release. The γ emission of Iodine-131 requires specific instructions to the Bexxar patient to sleep in a separate bed, not take a long trip, maintain >6 ft from others, avoid contact with children and pregnant women, etc.

MYCOSIS FUNGOIDES

General Principles

- Radiation therapy is indicated in the definitive management of localized disease and in symptomatic palliation of disseminated cutaneous, nodal, and/or visceral lesions.
  - Stage IA mycosis fungoides is most often treated locally with superficial electron beam radiation therapy.
  - For T2-T4 diseases, either multiple fields encompassing the main disease sites or total skin electron beam therapy (TSEBT) can be used as a primary treatment.

Localization, Immobilization, and Simulation

- Variable depending on the site being treated and on the type of treatment approach used.
- Total skin electron beam therapy will be discussed in a separate section.

Target Volumes and Organs of Interest Definition

- Stage IA mycosis fungoides.
    - Disease area with a 2- to 3-cm margin, ensuring coverage to a depth of 4 mm.
    - A single radiation field should be used whenever possible.
    - When matching fields due to size or geometric constraints, feathering of the field junctions should be done on a weekly basis to maximize dose homogeneity.
- Stage IB, II, and III mycosis fungoides
    - Multiple fields as defined in stage IA can be used to treat the main disease sites of more advanced disease.
    - TSEBT also used
        - Target volume of stage IB and II diseases to include the epidermis and dermis.
        - Target volume of stage III (cutaneous tumors) disease to include the full depth of the tumors.

Treatment Planning

Focal Therapy

- Usually, a clinical setup for en face electron fields, superficial x-ray units, or higher energy photons (ie, 6 MV) with bolus.

Critical Structures

- Clinical setup and technique will always take neighboring normal structures into account at the time of simulation (ie, skin folds, eyelid, etc), often resulting in complex clinical setups.

Technical Factors

Beam energies

- Selection based on tumor characteristics.
- Electron beam (6-12 MeV), superficial x-rays, or higher energy photons (ie, 6 MV) with bolus.

Beam shaping

■ Electron cutouts mounted on the corresponding cones are used for beam shaping.

Dose/Fractionation

■ Stage IA mycosis fungoides
  ■ Approximately 20 to 30 Gy in 1.8 to 2 Gy/fx.
  ■ Stage IB, II, and III mycosis fungoides:
    • When using multiple fields, the same guidelines as for stage IA apply.

Total Skin Electron Beam Therapy

■ Delivered over 9 weeks, 1 Gy per day, 4 days per week, with a 1-week break after week 4, to a total dose of 36 Gy (36 treatment days).
  ■ For TSEBT, 26 Gy or greater should be prescribed to a depth of 4 mm, with a surface dose of 31 to 36 Gy (4).

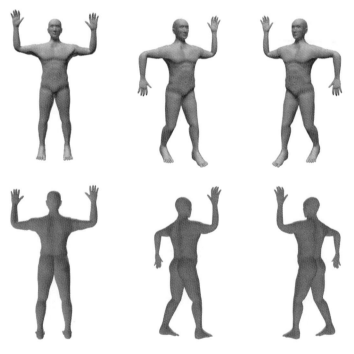

FIGURE 10.6 Six treatment positions used for total skin treatment: antero-posterior, right anterior oblique, left anterior oblique, posteroanterior, right posterior oblique, and left posterior oblique.

- A boost treatment to bulky or symptomatic areas 1 to 2 weeks prior to the delivery of TSEBT may be used.
  - 4 to 6 Gy in a single fraction, or 10 to 20 Gy in 5 to 10 fx, using en face electrons (energy dependent on target depth) with 1-cm margins.
- Six treatment positions ensure complete skin coverage (Figure 10.6).
- The treatment cycle consists of 3 of the 6 fields treated per day alternating over the 4 day weekly cycle.
  - The weekly schedule (only 4 treatment days) is AP/right posterior oblique/left posterior oblique on day 1 and PA/right anterior oblique/left anterior oblique on day 2, repeat for days 3 and 4.
  - This cycle is repeated 9 times.
- Each treatment position is treated with a split field to maximize dose homogeneity.
- Use nail and eye blocks to prevent overdosing these areas.
- In these treatment positions, the soles of the feet, scalp, inframammary, pannicular, perianal, buttocks/thighs, inner thighs, and perineal skin regions may be underdosed.
  - Some recommend patch treatment to the underdosed areas.

MULTIPLE MYELOMA/PLASMACYTOMA

General Principles

- EBRT only for palliation in the management of multiple myeloma.

Multiple Myeloma

- Palliative EBRT is indicated for pain related to bone or soft tissue disease, for neurological compromise, or for pathologic fracture or impending pathologic fracture after orthopedic stabilization. Radiation is usually given in a sequential fashion with relation to chemotherapy, as toxicity from concurrent treatment can be great.

Localization, Immobilization, and Simulation

- Variable depending on the site being treated. Usually, the patient is supine without any special immobilization, but proper reproducibility of setup in the target site is ensured.

Target Volumes and Organs of Interest Definition

- The radiographic lesion(s) plus a 2-cm margin. Coverage of the entire bone is not needed in long bones, except in cases where almost the entirety of the

bone would get treated otherwise and whole bone treatment would allow for easier field matches in the future.
- For vertebral lesions, the entire vertebra should be included with 1 or 2 vertebral bodies above and below.
- Hemibody radiation was used in the past for consolidation after chemotherapy but has now fallen out of favor.

Treatment Planning

Conventional treatment planning is sufficient for most of palliative treatments to long bones, usually with AP/PA field arrangement. In cases where there is soft tissue disease or nearby critical structures to be avoided, 3D CT–based treatment planning may be of use to more accurately define the treatment volume.

Critical Structures
- Doses used for treatment of myeloma rarely exceed normal tissue tolerance, and normal structures are not routinely delineated. For specific cases where tolerances could be exceeded, 3D treatment planning is done and structures are limited according to traditional dose constraints as explained elsewhere in this text.

Technical Factors

Beam energies
- Photon energies: 6 to 10 MV.

Beam shaping
- Multileaf collimation or individually shaped (5 HVL) custom blocks for normal tissue protection outside the target volume are used.

Dose/Fractionation
- The most commonly used dosing schemes for bone pain palliation (lower dose per fraction preferred for larger amounts of bowel or other sensitive structure in field) are 20 to 30 Gy in 5 to 15 fx (2-4 Gy/fx).
- In the setting of spinal cord compression caused by multiple myeloma, 30 Gy in 10 fx should be used.

SOLITARY PLASMACYTOMA OF BONE (OSSEOUS PLASMACYTOMA)

- Radiation therapy is the standard of care for solitary plasmacytoma of the bone, with surgery used for pathological fracture or stabilization of impending fractures and radiation given adjuvantly.

Localization, Immobilization, and Simulation

- Variable depending on the site being treated. Usually, the patient is supine without any special immobilization, but proper reproducibility of setup in the target site is ensured.

Target Volumes and Organs of Interest Definition

- The radiographic or clinically defined lesion(s) plus a 2- to 3-cm margin
  - For vertebral lesions, the entire vertebra should be included with 1 or 2 vertebral bodies above and below.

Treatment Planning

Therapy
- Conventional treatment planning is sufficient for the majority of treatments, usually with AP/PA field arrangement.
- Where there is soft tissue disease or nearby critical structures to be avoided, 3D CT–based treatment planning may be of use.

Critical Structures
- As a function of disease location and the dose used.

Technical Factors

Beam energies
- Photon energies: 6 to 10 MV.

Beam shaping
- Multlileaf collimation or individually shaped (5 HVL) custom blocks for normal tissue protection outside the target volume are used.

Dose/Fractionation
- Doses of 40 to 50 Gy/2 Gy/fx are the most frequently used regimens (5).

EXTRAMEDULLARY PLASMACYTOMA

- Radiation therapy is the standard of care for extramedullary plasmacytoma.

Localization, Immobilization, and Simulation

- Variable depending on the site being treated. Usually, the patient is supine without any special immobilization, but proper reproducibility of setup in the target site is ensured.

Target Volumes and Organs of Interest Definition

■ The radiographic or clinically defined lesion(s) plus a 2- to 3-cm margin.

Treatment Planning

Therapy

■ Conventional treatment planning is sufficient for the majority of treatments, usually with AP/PA field arrangement.
■ Where there is soft tissue disease or nearby critical structures to be avoided, 3D CT–based treatment planning may be of use.

Critical Structures

■ As a function of disease location and the dose used.

Technical Factors

Beam energies
■ Photon energies: 6 to 10 MV.

Beam shaping
■ Multlileaf collimation or individually shaped (5 HVL) custom blocks for normal tissue protection outside the target volume are used.

Dose/Fractionation
■ Doses of 40 to 50 Gy in 20 to 25 fx are the most frequently used regimens.
  ■ 50 Gy recommended for bulky disease.

TOTAL BODY IRRADIATION

General Principles

■ Used on its own, or as an adjunct to chemotherapy as part of a myeloablative regimen, to condition the host bone marrow prior to receiving a hematopoietic transplantation.

Localization, Immobilization, and Simulation

■ Variety of Total Body Irradiation (TBI) techniques.
■ Goal: to deliver low-dose rate RT (5-10 cGy/min) to a uniformity of ±10% to the midline at the umbillicus.
■ To achieve a 90% or higher surface dose, a 1- to 2-cm-thick acrylic is placed 10 cm in front of the patient (known as beam spoiler).

Opposed laterals technique

One needs to be aware of the lateral dose effect (ratio of D_{max} dose to mid-dose) due to the reduced thickness in the extremities.

- The patient is seated and treated with opposed lateral fields, using 10 MV photon beams and tissue compensators mounted on a tray to produce dose uniformity to within ±10% compared with prescription dose at midpoint at umbilicus.
- The patient's back is supported on the couch.
- Arms follow the body contour and shadow the lungs; however, using the arms to shield the lungs results in nonuniform dosimetry and compensators are recommended.

AP/PA technique

Provides better dose homogeneity and less need for tissue compensation (with the exception of lung blocks)

- The patient is in a standing position at 410 cm SAD pseudoisocentric AP/PA at the level of the umbilicus.
- 40 × 40 cm field with collimator rotated 45°.
- Harness and arm/leg rods assist in reproducibility.
- Partial transmission lung blocks are used to shield the lungs, screwed on to plastic supports close to the patient.
- Physician draws lung blocks on AP and PA films, with 1- to 1.5-cm margin around the lung border.
- Thickness of lung shielding variable: some institutions use 1 HVL throughout the treatment course, whereas others have used a single 7-HVL block for a single fraction only. With 1 HVL and other intermediate HVL values, Therma-Luminescent Dosimeter (TLD) dosimetry is performed with and without blocks to calculate the necessary number of blocked fractions for lungs to receive ~85% of prescribed dose.

Technical Factors

Beam energies
- Photon energies: 6 to 10 MV.

Beam shaping
- Cerrobend block used for lungs as "Localization, Immobilization, and Simulation" section.

Dose/Fractionation

- There is no standard treatment technique for TBI; significant differences in dose distributions exist with different treatment methods.
- Techniques include
  - AP/PA with a laying patient (supine and prone) being scanned through a fixed beam.
  - AP/PA with a laying patient (supine and prone) with rotating gantry head sweeping across the patient.
  - Arcs, helical tomotherapy, and others.
- Dose depends on institution, specific protocol, and indication but may vary from 4 Gy in 2 fx to 12 Gy in 6 to 8 fx.
- Testicles are boosted in male patients with leukemia, typically 4 Gy in 2 fx.

REFERENCES

1. Cheson BD, Horning SJ, Coiffier B, et al. Report of an international workshop to standardize response criteria for non-Hodgkin's lymphomas. NCI Sponsored International Working Group. *J Clin Oncol*. 1999;17:1244.

2. Juweid ME, Wiseman GA, Vose JM, et al. Response assessment of aggressive non-Hodgkin's lymphoma by integrated International Workshop Criteria and fluorine-18-fluorodeoxyglucose positron emission tomography. *J Clin Oncol*. 2005;23:4652–4661.

3. Yahalom J, Mauch P. The involved field is back: issues in delineating the radiation field in Hodgkin's disease. *Ann Oncol*. 2002;13(Suppl 1):79–83.

4. Jones GW, Kacinski BM, Wilson LD, et al. Total skin electron radiation in the management of mycosis fungoides: consensus of the European Organization for Research and Treatment of Cancer (EORTC) Cutaneous Lymphoma Project Group. *J Am Acad Dermatol*. 2002;47:364–370.

5. Knobel D, Zouhair A, Tsang RW, et al. Prognostic factors in solitary plasmacytoma of the bone: a multicenter Rare Cancer Network study. *BMC Cancer* 2006;6:118.

11 Soft Tissue Sarcoma Radiotherapy

Grant K. Hunter, Andrew D. Vassil, Abigail L. Stockham, Samuel T. Chao, and Gregory M. M. Videtic

GENERAL PRINCIPLES

- Surgical resection is the foundation of sarcoma treatment.
- External beam radiation (EBRT) and brachytherapy techniques are used in the preoperative and postoperative settings for the extremities and in the retroperitoneum.

Localization, Immobilization, and Simulation

- Localization
  - Spiral computed tomography (CT) with 3-mm slices spanning the target region.
  - Large bore scanner gives maximum flexibility in arranging the limb so that the contralateral extremity and trunk are out of the beam.
  - Contrast is not typically used.
- Immobilization

- Positioning is highly dependent on the site.
- Most patients are positioned supine; the affected extremities are positioned to maximize reproducibility and treatment angle options while minimizing exposure to adjacent structures.
- Vacuum-locking bags and body molds aid in making positioning reproducible.
- Simulation
    - Radiopaque wires are used to mark biopsy site (preoperative) or surgical incision (postoperative).
    - Isocenter is placed at least D_{max} depth from the surface and typically in a central location within the anticipated treatment volume.

Target Volumes and Organs of Interest Definition

- Knowledge of muscle compartments and fascial planes is mandatory for appropriate treatment planning.
- Target volumes may include gross disease, tumor bed, and surgical scar.
- Dose-limiting normal structures vary depending on site and should be delineated on planning CT if located near the target volumes.
- Surrounding normal structures are delineated for dose assessment at the time of treatment planning.
- Preoperative and postoperative diagnostic imaging studies are used to aid in target localization.

Treatment Planning

- For both EBRT and brachytherapy, CT-based 3-dimensional planning is favored over 2-dimensional planning to reduce normal tissue dose and better delineate target area.
- IMRT and image-guided radiation therapy are exploratory and not standard in this setting.
- Dose distribution are calculated with heterogeneity correction and reviewed on all images.

Critical Structures

- Critical structures are site dependent.
    - For extremities, joint spaces and bone are typically in or near treatment volumes. A strip of skin is spared to limit the risk of lymphedema.
    - For retroperitoneal sarcomas, the spinal cord, bowel, kidneys, and bladder may be in or near treatment volumes.
- Coverage of the PTV to control disease takes priority; however, limiting dose to normal tissues should be attempted.

- Less than 50% of a longitudinal strip of skin and subcutaneous tissue to 20 Gy.
- Avoid full prescription dose to the skin over areas commonly traumatized (elbow, knee, and shin).
- Less than 50% normal weight-bearing bone to 50 Gy except if involved with tumor.
- Less than 50% femoral head/neck to 60 Gy.
- Less than 50% any joint to 50 Gy.
- Less than 50% anus and vulva to 30 Gy.
- Less than 50% testis to 3 Gy.
- V20 lung ≤37%.

Technical Factors

- For the extremities, 6-MV photons are favored because higher energy beams may underdose superficial tissues.
- Bolus is applied to surgical scars to increase skin dose.
- Dose homogeneity may be improved with tissue compensators (including physical wedges, dynamic wedges, segmented field technique, and IMRT) and supplementation with higher energy beams.

EXTREMITY SARCOMA EBRT

Introduction

- Preoperative versus postoperative EBRT are both used, as there are benefits and complications associated with each. Clinical presentations will favor one over the other.

Localization, Immobilization, and Simulation

- When treating an extremity, immobilization of the joints distal and proximal to the target aids in reproducing setup (Figure 11.1a).

Target Volumes and Organs of Interest Definition

- Soft tissue sarcomas (STS) are generally surrounded by a region of compressed reactive tissue that forms a pseudocapsule, followed by a reactive zone (high T2 signal on MRI) that can harbor microscopic disease.
- Preoperative MRI (T1 with contrast, T2) is necessary for target definition in both the preoperative and postoperative settings.
- Postoperative MRI may be helpful after surgery to identify regions of suspected gross residual tumor.

FIGURE 11.1 Patient with synovial cell sarcoma of the right proximal gastrocnemius. The patient was positioned prone with the left leg "frog-legged" out on a vacuum locking cradle device for CT simulation (a). Using a coregistered MRI for target delineation (b), a 4-field plan with 6-MV photons (c) was used to deliver 50 Gy to the 96.5% IDL (d). Image guidance using kV-cone-beam CT was used for daily localization (e). Wedges were used for the lateral beams, and beams were weighted 3:2, favoring lateral beams.

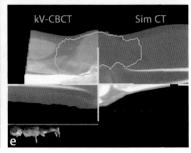

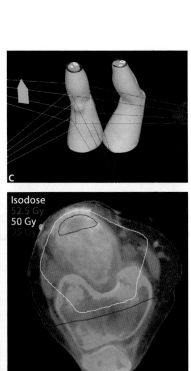

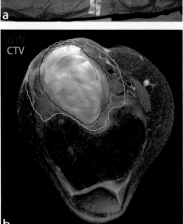

- Modified from O'Sullivan et al (1), to include use of MRI to define "tissues at risk".
- Select portions of the margins may be reduced if the tumor is confined by an intact fascial barrier, bone, or skin surface. Note that margins are classically block margins.
- Preoperative radiotherapy (RT)
  - GTV = gross tumor defined by MRI T1 plus contrast.
  - CTV = GTV + suspicious edema defined by MRI T2 + 5-cm longitudinal margins and 2-cm radial margins.
  - PTV = CTV + error for setup and organ motion, typically 0.5 to 1 cm.
- Postoperative RT
  - Metallic clips or gold seeds placed during surgery aid in defining the tumor bed.
  - GTV = gross tumor defined by MRI T1 plus contrast.
  - CTV1 = GTV + suspicious edema defined by MRI T2 + 5-cm longitudinal margins and 2-cm radial margins.
  - CTV2 = GTV + 2 cm.
  - PTV = CTV + error for setup and organ motion, typically 0.5 to 1 cm.
- Organs of interest include the skin, bone, and joints; testes and ovaries may be considered during treatment planning for proximal thigh lesions.

Treatment Planning

- The minimum dose to a point within the PTV is 97% of the prescription dose, and 95% of the PTV is covered with that prescription dose. No more than 20% of the PTV receives a dose that is 110% or higher the prescribed dose (Figure 11.1b).
- 3-Dimensional conformal RT
  - For distal extremity lesions, opposed lateral fields and multifield arrangements, with wedges to compensate for changes in extremity thickness (Figure 11.1c).
  - More proximal structures often require more complex field arrangements, wedging, and IMRT.
  - Planning target volume margins may be reduced with the use of image-guided RT (Figure 11.1d).

Dose/Fractionation

- Preoperative RT
  - 50 Gy/2 Gy/fx to PTV
  - 44 Gy/2 Gy/fx to the PTV if concurrent or interdigitated chemotherapy is used. Interdigitated chemotherapy is typically delivered after 22 Gy (11 fx).

- Add postoperative boost of 16 Gy for microscopically positive margins and 25 Gy for gross residual disease.
- Postoperative RT
  - 50 Gy in 25 fx to PTV1, followed by a boost to PTV2 to 60 Gy for negative margins, 66 Gy for microscopically positive margins, 75 Gy for gross residual.

Intraoperative Boost

- Electron beam therapy may be used in the intraoperative setting to deliver 10 to 12.5 Gy in 1 fx to an area microscopically positive at the time of resection (documented by frozen section).
- Electron energy is typically chosen such that a 1-cm depth or 90% isodose line covers the desired treatment area.

EXTREMITY SARCOMA—BRACHYTHERAPY

Introduction

- Brachytherapy techniques include postoperative low-dose rate or high-dose rate using implanted catheters and other temporary applicators.
- For patients with intermediate to high grade with either positive or negative margins, brachytherapy can be used to boost wide-field EBRT.

Localization, Immobilization, and Simulation

- Metallic clips or gold seeds are recommended to be placed during surgery to aid in defining the residual tumor bed for a positive margin.

Target Volumes and Organs of Interest Definition

- CTV = tumor bed visualized on imaging studies and under direct inspection intraoperatively.
- The American Brachytherapy Society (2) recommends an at least 2- to 5-cm longitudinal margin beyond CTV and 1- to 2-cm spacing between catheters.

Treatment Planning

- HDR brachytherapy catheters are implanted approximately 1 cm apart along the tumor bed, and radio-opaque clips indicate the margins. Optimized treatment planning can be used to deliver a more homogeneous dose.
- In most cases, a single plane implant will be sufficient to cover the CTV.

- Nerve tolerance to high dose per fraction is poor, and HDR should be used with caution when catheters have to be placed in contact with neurovascular structures.
- American Brachytherapy Society guidelines to minimize morbidity with brachytherapy (2).
  - When brachytherapy is used as adjuvant monotherapy, the source loading should start no sooner than 5 to 6 days after wound closure. However, the radioactive sources may be loaded earlier (as soon as 2-3 days after surgery) if doses of less than 20 Gy are given with brachytherapy as a supplement to EBRT.
  - Minimize dose to normal tissues (eg, gonads, breasts, thyroid, and skin) whenever possible, especially in children and patients of childbearing age.
  - Limit the allowable skin dose: the 40-Gy isodose line (LDR) to less than 25 cm and the 25-Gy isodose line to less than 100 cm^2.

Dose/Fractionation

- In general, the dose delivered is related to the dose rate and whether EBRT is used.
- Prescription point is usually 5 to 10 mm from the plane of the implant.

If using

- LDR monotherapy: 45 to 50 Gy/4 to 6 days, ~0.45 Gy/h.
- LDR with EBRT: 15 to 25 Gy/2 to 3 days, ~0.45 Gy/h.
- HDR fractionated: 32 to 50 Gy/4 to 7 days, twice daily every 6 hours.
- HDR with EBRT: 12 to 18 Gy/3 days, twice daily every 6 hours.

Doses of 40 to 50 Gy are given in 12 to 15 fx if the HDR is given alone. If EBRT (45-50 Gy) is added, the brachytherapy dose is limited to 18 to 25 Gy in 4 to 7 fx.

RETROPERITONEAL SARCOMA—EBRT AND BRACHYTHERAPY

Introduction

- Radiotherapy may be given either preoperatively or postoperatively.
- Preoperative RT offers several theoretical and practical advantages over postoperative therapy (Figure 11.2).
  - Optimal knowledge of the extent of disease is possible for treatment planning.
  - Radiotherapy morbidity is usually less.
  - Tumor bulk displaces dose-limiting small bowel.

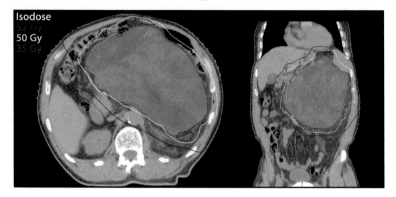

FIGURE 11.2 Patient with a dedifferentiated liposarcoma of the abdomen. Patient was positioned supine, and IMRT planning using 8 fields of 6-MV photons prescribed to the 98% isodose line was used to deliver 50 Gy preoperative RT; daily IGRT was performed with cone-beam CT.

- The bowel is unlikely to be fixed by surgical adhesions seen postoperatively.
- Potentially smaller portal is needed as compared with postoperative RT when trying to cover surgically manipulated tissue.
- There is a possibility for increased complete resection rate secondary to tumor shrinkage.
- Risk of intraperitoneal tumor dissemination may be reduced.
- Intact peritoneal covering provides a physical barrier to early tumor dissemination.
- Displaced normal tissue may permit dose escalation.
- Radiobiologic advantage of intact vascularity and, thus, less tissue hypoxia as in the postoperative setting.
- Disadvantages of preoperative RT include the following:
  - Compromised wound healing after surgery.
  - Delay in surgical resection.
  - Accurate staging may be compromised.

Localization, Immobilization, and Simulation

- Metallic clips or gold seeds are recommended to be placed during surgery to aid in defining the residual tumor bed for a positive margin for intraoperative and postoperative RT.

- Saline-filled tissue expander placed at time of resection is safe and may reduce morbidity (3).

Target Volumes and Organs of Interest Definition

- GTV equals the imaging defined tumor.
- CTV is a 1- to 2-cm margin on GTV.
- PTV expansions are specific to institutional and patient setup parameters.

Treatment Planning

- IMRT may be particularly appropriate, given the range of normal tissues.
- One kidney commonly is within the PTV.
  - Always document the function of the contralateral kidney.
  - Determine the total renal function to ensure adequate residual renal function.
- Normal tissue toxicities of relevance (Table 11.1).

Dose/Fractionation

- Base preoperative /postoperative dose: 45 to 50 Gy/1.8 Gy/fx.
- In the postoperative setting, consider an EBRT beam boost of 5.4 to 9 Gy as deemed safe (Figure 11.3).
- Option as available: intraoperative boost of 10 to 15 Gy using electron-beam therapy or brachytherapy (Figure 11.4).

TABLE 11.1 Retroperitoneal Sarcoma—External Beam Radiotherapy and Brachytherapy: Normal Tissue Toxicities of Relevance

Organ\Fraction of organ	1/3	2/3	3/3	End Point
Stomach	60 Gy	55 Gy	50 Gy	Ulceration/perforation
Kidneys	50 Gy	30 Gy	23 Gy	Nephritis
Liver	90 Gy	47 Gy	31 Gy	Liver failure
Small intestine	50 Gy	–	40 Gy	Obstruction/fistula/perforation
Colon	55 Gy	–	45 Gy	Obstruction/fistula/perforation

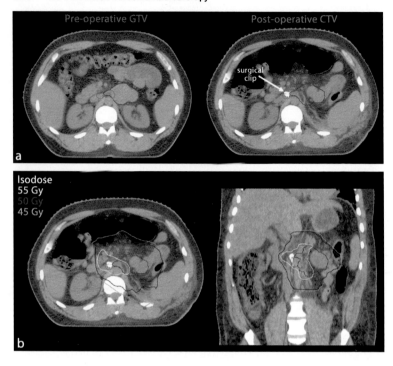

FIGURE 11.3 Patient with resected retroperitoneal leiomyosarcoma. Preoperative CT images were coregistered with the simulation CT to aid in target localization (a). IMRT planning using 5 fields of 10-MV photons prescribed to the 98% isodose line was used to deliver 55 Gy to the postoperative CTV (b); daily IGRT was performed with cone-beam CT.

FIGURE 11.4 Patient with leiomyosarcoma of the retroperitoneum. After en bloc tumor resection, the tumor bed received 28 Gy in 4 fx of 7 Gy (>6-hour interfraction interval) prescribed to the 100% isodose line at a depth of 0.5 cm using a Harrison-Anderson-Mick (HAM) applicator. Bowel and abdominal wall was displaced with sterile temporary packing.

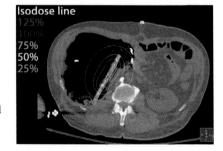

HETEROTOPIC OSSIFICATION

RT Indications

- Perioperatively for patients who have undergone orthopedic intervention with a history of prior heterotopic ossification, diffuse idiopathic skeletal hyperostosis, and hypertrophic osteoarthritis, particularly for patients in whom medical treatment with indomethacin is not an option.
- Treat less than 24 hours preoperatively or less than 72 hours postoperatively.

Localization, Immobilization, Simulation

- Positioning: supine with the area to be treated isolated as much as possible (eg, for elbow, may consider arms akimbo).
- Localization: at the site of surgical intervention.
- Immobilization: no formal immobilization techniques are used.
- Simulation: CT simulation, although fluoroscopic simulation is feasible.
- Planning: typically, anteroposterior/posteroanterior fields with dose prescribed to midplane.

Volumes, Dose, and Fractionation

- Volumes (Figure 11.5)
  - Include soft tissue surrounding the joint space.
  - Field size is approximately 7 × 12 cm for the hip.
  - Role of blocking surgical hardware is controversial.

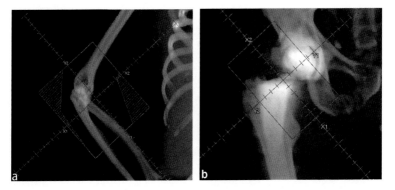

FIGURE 11.5 Treatment fields from patients with resected heterotopic ossification of the elbow (a) and right hip (b).

- Dose and fractionation
  - 7 Gy in 1 fx via anteroposterior/posteroanterior fields with 10 to 18 MV photons.

REFERENCES

1. O'Sullivan B, Davis AM, Turcotte R, et al. Preoperative versus postoperative radiotherapy in soft-tissue sarcoma of the limbs: a randomised trial. *Lancet.* 2002;359:2235–2241.

2. Nag S, Shasha D, Janjan N, Petersen I, Zaider M. The American Brachytherapy Society recommendations for brachytherapy of soft tissue sarcomas. *Int J Radiat Oncol Biol Phys.* 2001;49:1033–1043.

3. White JS, Biberdorf D, DiFrancesco LM, Kurien E, Temple W. Use of tissue expanders and pre-operative external beam radiotherapy in the treatment of retroperitoneal sarcoma. *Ann Surg Oncol.* 2007;14:583–590.

12 Pediatric Radiotherapy

Erin S. Murphy, Lawrence J. Sheplan,
and Samuel T. Chao

INTRODUCTION

- There are approximately 12,000 cases of pediatric malignancies per year.
- The most common include leukemia, CNS malignancies, and lymphoma.
- Radiotherapy plays an important role in children with solid tumors and, to a lesser extent, childhood leukemia.
- This chapter will focus on photon-based EBRT. Proton therapy is an option for pediatric malignancies and is currently being investigated at several institutions.

General Principles

- Radiotherapy can affect the development and growth of normal tissues. Because of the young age of children at the time of treatment, understanding normal tissue treatment effects is paramount and techniques should be used to minimize the long-term toxicities.
- Specific dose prescription will be determined by tumor types and treatment approaches, such as, preoperative, definitive, or postoperative therapy.

Localization, Immobilization, and Simulation

- Most children younger than 5 years will require daily anesthesia.
  - Techniques include conscious sedation, deep sedation, or general anesthesia.
- Behavioral techniques such as talking with the child via a microphone in the console room or playing a video in the treatment room may facilitate simulation and treatment without anesthesia for cooperative children.
- A pretreatment tour of the simulation and treatment rooms may facilitate a better experience for the patient and family.
- Patient positioning will depend on the treatment site.
- CT simulation +/- IV contrast will enable 3D treatment planning for definition of GTV, CTV, and PTV.
- Immobilization: devices such as thermoplastic mesh for head masks, supine and prone head holders, or vacuum locking (vac-loc) bags allow for easily customizable immobilization.
  - Planning target volume margins should take the degree of immobilization into account.
  - Angled knee sponges and banding of feet aid in reproducing set-up.
  - Special care must be given to working with the anesthesia team for safety of the patient during treatment, with attention to the airway, IV access, and monitors.
- Contiguous spiral CT slices with 3-mm slice acquisition to include the entire treatment volume plus margin. The scan should also include normal tissue structures that are to be contoured.
- Localization: an isocenter should be placed in the middle of the target volume.
  - Information from operative reports, preoperative and postoperative iodine-131-meta-iodobenzylguanidine (MIBG) scintiscan MRI/CT scan, and PET studies may be incorporated to aid in target localization.

Target Volumes and Organs of Interest Definition

- For help delineating target volumes, one may reference the current Children's Oncology Group (COG) protocol for guidance.
- Structures of interest should be identified and depend on the location of the tumor.
  - Brain: lens, eyes, optic nerves, optic chiasm, pituitary, hypothalamus, brainstem, cochlea, temporal lobes, spinal cord, and cribriform fossa (for whole-brain EBRT).
  - Spine: spinal cord, thyroid, and male or female sex organs.

- Abdomen: kidneys, spinal cord, liver, male or female sex organs, and small bowel.
- Chest: lungs, heart, spinal cord, esophagus, liver, and kidneys.

WILMS TUMOR

RT Indications

- The National Wilms Tumor Studies have developed a multidisciplinary treatment approach that involves upfront surgical staging followed by chemotherapy and radiotherapy when necessary.
- In general, EBRT is not indicated for stage I and II tumors, unless they are unfavorable histologies.
- Regardless of histology, EBRT is indicated for stage III and IV.

Localization, Immobilization, and Simulation

- Positioning: patient should be in supine position with arms above the head or akimbo especially if lung radiotherapy is necessary.
- Localization: use operative reports and preoperative imaging to delineate operative bed and/or residual disease.
- Immobilization: a device such as a vac-loc bag aids in reproducing set-up.
- Simulation: A 4D or fluoroscopic simulation should be used to determine the extent of motion of the targets and organs at risk, with particular attention regarding the lungs.

RT Indication and Dose/Fractionation

Special Considerations
- Radiotherapy to begin by postoperative day 9.
- Dose per fraction is 1.8 Gy, except when large volumes are receiving EBRT in which case the dose is reduced to 1.5 Gy.
- For patients 16 years or older, 30.6 Gy is prescribed for bone, lymph node, and brain metastases; 19.8 Gy should be delivered to the flank or abdomen.
- Any stage patient with clear cell sarcoma of the kidney should receive 10.8 Gy per the stage III field indications (although stage I is controversial).
- Any stage patient with rhabdoid tumor should receive 19.8 Gy per the stage III field indications. Consider a lower dose for children younger than 1 year.
- For stage V patients, preoperative chemotherapy is usually given. Each tumor should be staged separately. Flank EBRT is recommended for patients with positive margins or positive nodes to a dose of 10.8 Gy. Whole abdominal

TABLE 12.1 Wilms Tumor: EBRT Indication and Dose/Fractionation

Stage	Histology	EBRT Indicated	EBRT Field	EBRT Dose
I	FH	No		
	UH	Yes	Flank	10.8/1.8 Gy/fx
II	FH	No		
	UH	Yes	Flank	10.8 Gy
III	FH	Yes	Flank: surgical spillage, flank or peritoneal biopsy, open biopsy.	Flank: 10.8 Gy
	UH	Yes		
			WAI (whole abdominal EBRT): cytology + ascites, preoperative tumor rupture, diffuse abdominal surgical spillage, peritoneal seeding	WAI: 10.5 Gy except for diffuse unresectable peritoneal implants: 21 Gy/1.5 Gy/fx
IV	FH/UH	Yes	WLI (whole lung EBRT): lung metastases	12 Gy/1.5 Gy/fx; 10.5 Gy for age <12 y
			Whole brain plus boost : brain metastases	21.6 Gy+ boost of 10.8 Gy
			Whole/partial liver: liver metastases	19.8 Gy
			Partial bone: bone metastases	25.2 Gy
			Lymph nodes (unresected)	19.8 Gy
V	FH/UH	Depends on individual tumor stage	Flank: +margins or +LN	10.8 Gy
			WAI: as per stage III indications (Consider smaller field for renal sparing as per COG)	10.5 Gy

Abbreviations: COG, Children's Oncology Group; FH, favorable histology; UH, unfavorable histology; WAI, whole abdominal irradiation; WLI, whole lung irradiation.

EBRT is required as per stage III indications above to a dose of 10.5 Gy. Gross disease should receive a boost of 10.8 Gy. For special considerations of small field renal sparing radiotherapy, see the COG protocols.

- Boost gross residual disease that is greater than 3 cm with an additional 10.8 Gy.
- For diffuse anaplasia, a dose of 19.8 to 20 Gy should be used.
- Irradiating lung metastases is controversial when diagnosed on chest CT or when there is favorable histology or complete response to chemotherapy.
- Persistent focal lung disease 2 weeks after whole lung irradiation (WLI) should be excised or receive a boost of 7.5 Gy in 5 fx.

Target Volumes and Treatment Planning

- If WLI and flank or whole abdominal irradiation (WAI) are required, then the fields can be treated simultaneously or sequentially. If treating simultaneously, the dose per fraction should be reduced to 1.5 Gy. If treating sequentially, typically treat WLI first. In some cases, both the lung and abdomen/flank can be treated with 1 field. If the areas are treated with 2 separate fields, the match line should be feathered to prevent excess liver and kidney dose. The match line should be moved by 0.5 cm in one direction approximately every few Gy (Figure 12.1).
- WLI (AP/PA): both lungs are targeted regardless of the location/number of metastases. A 1-cm margin should be added around the entire external pleural surface (Figure 12.2).

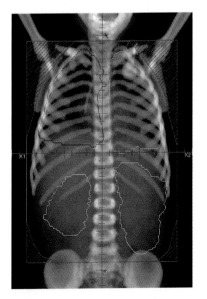

FIGURE 12.1 A 4-year-old with bilateral Wilms tumor, stage V, with bilateral pulmonary metastases s/p chemotherapy and right partial nephrectomy and resection of lymph nodes. Treatment: 10.5 Gy/1.5 Gy/ fx to bilateral lungs and bilateral flank delivered via AP/PA fields using 6 MV-photons. Lung and bilateral kidneys are contoured.

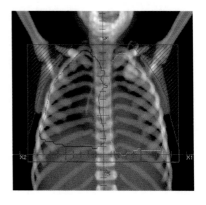

FIGURE 12.2 The bilateral lungs received an additional 1.5 Gy in 1 fx, for a total dose of 12 Gy. Right lung contour in blue, left in green.

■ Flank (AP/PA): the tumor and involved kidney as determined by the pre-operative CT scan is the GTV. A 1- to 2-cm margin should be added for the CTV; however, if the medial border extends to a vertebral body then the CTV needs to include the entire body plus a margin of 1 cm (Figures 12.3 and 12.4).

■ WAI (AP/PA): the superior border is 1 cm above the diaphragm; inferior border is at the bottom of the obturator foramen (with the femoral heads blocked) and the lateral borders are 1 cm beyond the lateral abdominal walls. 3DCRT or IMRT may be used to boost gross residual disease.

■ Whole brain: opposed laterals. For patients who receive a dose of 21.6 Gy and have 3 or more lesions, a boost of 10.8 Gy may be given by IMRT or single-fraction SRS.

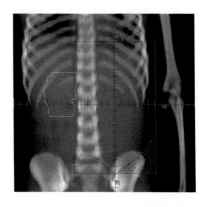

FIGURE 12.3 A 5-year-old with stage I Wilms tumor with diffuse anaplasia, s/p resection. The flank was treated to 10.8 Gy/1.8 Gy/fx via AP/PA techniques using 6-MV photons prescribed to the 98% IDL. The contralateral kidney is contoured in green.

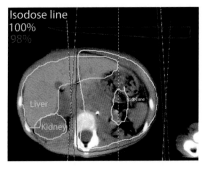

FIGURE 12.4 Axial CT slice of the plan from Figure 12.3 demonstrating the 100% IDL (yellow) and the 98% IDL (blue). The dose was prescribed to the 98% IDL for optimal coverage of the vertebral body.

- Liver: for diffuse disease, the entire liver is the target. Otherwise, the lesions as seen on imaging plus a 2-cm margin comprise the target. Of note, if the lesion is solitary and resected with negative margins, radiotherapy is not indicated.
- Lymph nodes: the metastatic lymph nodes as determined by the pretreatment imaging comprise the GTV. A 2-cm margin is added for the CTV.
- Bone metastases: the bone lesion as seen on CT or MRI will determine the GTV and a 3-cm margin is added for the CTV.

TABLE 12.2 Wilms Tumor: Normal Tissue Tolerance (per COG protocols)

Structure	Dose Limit, Gy
Small bowel	45
Spinal cord	45
Lung (<50% of the volume is included)	18
Lung (>50% of the volume is included)	15
Kidney (WAI dose >10.5, shield the normal kidney to ≤14.4 Gy)	19.8
Whole liver	23.4

Abbreviations: COG, Children's Oncology Group; WAI, whole abdominal irradiation.

NEUROBLASTOMA

RT Indications

- High-risk patients: used to treat primary tumor site and persistent metastatic sites as seen on MIBG scan.
- Intermediate-risk patients: for recurrent/gross residual disease.

- Low-risk patients: not indicated after STR or gross total resection.
- For palliation in stage 4S disease, given to the liver if there is respiratory compromise from rapid hepatomegaly, especially in very young (1-2 months old) patients.

Localization, Immobilization, and Simulation

- Positioning: the patient should be in supine position with arms above the head or akimbo, especially if lung radiotherapy is necessary.
- Localization: use operative reports and preoperative imaging to delineate operative bed and/or residual disease.
- Immobilization: a device such as a vac-loc bag aids in reproducing set-up.
- Simulation: a 4D or fluoroscopic simulation should be used to determine the extent of motion of the targets and organs at risk, with particular attention regarding the lungs.

Target Volumes and Dose

- GTV: the tumor and positive nodal disease as determined by the preoperative CT scan and operative report. A 1- to 2-cm margin should be added for the CTV; however, if the border extends to a vertebral body, then the CTV needs to include the entire body plus a margin of 1 cm (Figure 12.5).
- Dose
  - 21.6 Gy/1.8 Gy/fx daily (COG).
  - 21 Gy/1.5 Gy/fx twice daily (Memorial Sloan-Kettering Cancer Center [MSKCC]).
  - St Jude protocol NB2005 prescribed 23.4 Gy to microscopic and 30.6 Gy to gross disease.
- Palliative liver: 4.5 Gy/1.5 Gy/fx.
- Critical structures (Table 12.3).

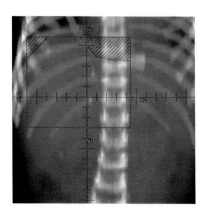

FIGURE 12.5 A 3-year-old with neuroblastoma, stage IV, s/p induction chemotherapy and resection (tumor crosses midline, N-myc+, LN+, negative margins after neoadjuvant chemotherapy) and consolidative radiotherapy to the primary disease per COG A3973 protocol. The primary tumor plus a 2-cm margin received 21.6 Gy/1.8 Gy/fx, prescribed to the midplane and delivered with 6-MV photons. COG indicates Children's Oncology Group.

TABLE 12.3 Neuroblastoma: Critical Structures

Organ	Dose Constraint
Liver	≤50% to receive >9 Gy and ≤25% to receive >18 Gy
Contralateral kidney	≤50% to receive >8 Gy and ≤20% to receive >12 Gy
Heart	100% to receive ≤20 Gy and 50% to receive ≤25 Gy
Lung	1/3 to receive ≥15 Gy
Ovaries	Block when possible; consider transposition

Treatment Planning

■ Three-dimensional imaging should be used to delineate the target and the normal tissue volumes.
■ Beam arrangement: simple AP/PA or 3D planning may be used.

RHABDOMYOSARCOMA

RT Indications (Table 12.4)

■ Not indicated for group I embryonal.
■ Adjuvant radiotherapy for group I alveolar/undifferentiated and all group II patients.
■ Definitive radiotherapy for all group III patients.
■ Curative intent radiotherapy to primary and metastatic sites (except bone marrow) for group IV.

Localization, Immobilization, and Simulation

■ Positioning: dependent on site of primary
  ■ For head and neck sites, the patient should be supine with the neck extended.

TABLE 12.4 Rhabdomyosarcoma: IRS Clinical Group Classification

IRS Clinical Group Classification	
Group I	Localized disease, completely resected
Group II	+ microscopic residual or + Regional LN completely resected
Group III	Gross residual after biopsy/resection
Group IV	Distant metastases

Abbreviation: IRS, Intergroup Rhabdomyosarcoma Study.

- For extremities, the patient should be positioned in such a way to enable a beam arrangement that would avoid normal tissues and spare a strip of skin.
- Localization: use operative reports and preoperative imaging to delineate operative bed and/or residual disease.
- Immobilization: a device such as a vac-loc bag aids in reproducible daily set-up. A bite block should be used when treating a head and neck site.
- Simulation: a CT simulation should be performed for 3D planning.

Target Volumes and Dose

- GTV: the tumor and positive nodal disease as determined by the preoperative CT/MRI scan, operative report, and radiopaque clips placed intraoperatively. A 1- to 2-cm margin should be added for the CTV, unless when using daily image guidance which would allow for margin reduction.
- If initial disease responded to chemotherapy and allowed for normal anatomy to resume its natural position, treat initially involved parenchyma but shave CTV off initially uninvolved tissue (eg, lung/bowel) that has returned to normal location and is now in the treatment field.
- Dose (Table 12.5)
- Critical structures (Table 12.6)
- Special considerations
  - Orbit: biopsy alone is sufficient. GTV + 5 mm PTV margin to 45 Gy for group III. Orbital exenteration for salvage only. The patient should be treated with the eye open unless the eyelid is involved.
  - Parameningeal: radiotherapy is given first if there is intracranial extension. The volume is the tumor as seen on MRI + 2-cm margin. Whole brain is used for extensive parenchymal involvement.
  - Vagina and vulva: resection followed by chemotherapy and second look surgery at week 12 (vulvar) or week 28 (vaginal). Complete vaginectomy

TABLE 12.5 Rhabdomyosarcoma: Dose

Group	Histology	Lymph Nodes	Dose, Gy
I	Poor	–	36 (IRSV) or 41.4
II	Good	Negative	36 (IRSV)
	Good	Positive	41.4
	Poor	–	41.4
III	–	–	50.4 (may cone down at 36 or 41.4)
IV	–	–	50. 4 (primary and metastatic sites)

Abbreviations: IRSV, Intergroup Rhabdomyosarcoma Study Group V.

TABLE 12.6 Rhabdomyosarcoma: Critical Structures

Organ	Dose Limit, Gy
Kidney	14.4
Whole liver	23.4
Bilateral lungs	15 (1.5 Gy/fx)
Whole brain ≥3 y old	30.6
<3 y old	23.4
Optic nerve and chiasm	46.8
Spinal cord	45
Gastrointestinal tract (partial)	45
Whole abdomen/pelvis	24 (1.5 Gy/fx)
Whole heart	30.6
Lens	14.4
Lacrimal gland/cornea	41.4

is inappropriate unless there is persistent/recurrent disease. If pathologic complete response (pCR) is noted from biopsy, no further treatment. If biopsy is positive, resect. If unresectable, use radiotherapy either by external beam or brachytherapy.

■ Testicular: inguinal orchiectomy and resection of spermatic cord and retroperitoneal lymph node dissection (RPLND) if there are involved nodes on CT or the patient is older than 10 years. RPLND is controversial in the absence of positive lymph nodes (+LN) on imaging studies. Radiotherapy to hemiscrotum, or hemiscrotectomy if the scrotum is violated.

■ Bladder: chemoradiotherapy for organ preservation when possible, followed by aggressive surgery for residual or progressive disease.

■ Extremity: a 2-cm margin around the mass or tumor bed as defined by MRI. Lymph nodes are treated only when involved. A strip of skin should be spared.

■ Thorax: any pulmonary metastases or pleural effusion receive whole lung RT 15 Gy in 1.5 Gy/fx (AP/PA fields); boost residual lung disease (if only a few nodules are present) to 50.4 Gy with 3D-CRT. (See WLI figure in "Wilms Tumor" section.)

■ Reproductive organs:
  • For males, consider transposition of contralateral testicle to the thigh before EBRT if scrotal EBRT is required.
  • Consider sperm banking when male is of reproductive age and expected fractionated dose to testes exceeds 2.5 to 3 Gy.

- For females, consider ovarian transposition to block from EBRT. Permanent sterility is age and dose dependent: 12 Gy for prepuberty and 2 Gy for premenopausal.

Treatment Planning

- Three-dimensional imaging should be used to delineate the target and the normal tissue volumes.
- Beam arrangement: depends on the primary site. The use of 3D conformal planning is recommended.
  - Pelvic sites: 4-field box, arcs, AP/PA (spares femoral epiphyseal plates and proximal femurs), or IMRT.

RETINOBLASTOMA

RT Treatment Options

- Radioactive plaques: solitary 2- to 16-mm basal diameter unilateral lesions located more than 3 mm from the optic disk or fovea, less than 10 mm thick, and for local failure after other therapy.
- EBRT: bilateral tumors, multifocal tumors, tumor location close to the macula or optic nerve, and preserved vision.

Plaque Brachytherapy Technique

- Plaque isotopes include ^{60}Co, ^{125}I, ^{192}Ir, and ^{109}Ru (not FDA approved). The different isotopes provide different isodose distributions and ^{125}I and ^{192}Ir have replaced ^{60}Co.
  - ^{125}I is the preferred isotope in the United States and Canada.
    - ^{125}I physical properties: half-life of 59 days, 28-keV γ-ray energy, and half-value layer of 0.025 mm of lead.
    - Plaques are typically made of gold and range from 10 to 22 mm in diameter.
    - Plaques can be customized according to the tumor shape or location by gluing the ^{125}I seeds to the concave surface of the plaque.
  - Dose: 40 to 45 Gy to the tumor apex, typically delivered over 48 to 96 hours (Figure 12.6); 25 to 30 Gy is recommended after chemotherapy.
- The procedure is performed under general anesthesia.
  - After the conjunctiva is opened, the tumor location is identified by using a transilluminator placed on the globe and then confirmed by indirect ophthalmoscopic globe depression.
  - An inactive plaque is placed with loose sutures in the exact location and is then replaced by the active plaque, which is sutured to the sclera and the conjunctiva is closed.

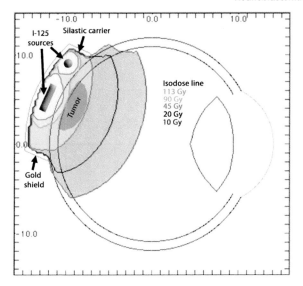

FIGURE 12.6 ^{125}I plaque demonstrating 45 Gy coverage of the tumor outlined in green.

- ▪ A lead shield is placed over a patch in front of the eye.
- ▪ The patient is brought back to the operating room under general anesthesia for removal of the plaque after the prescribed dose has been delivered.
- ▪ RT precautions
  - While the plaque is in place, the patient is kept in the hospital and advised to wear the lead eye shield.
  - The patient's body receives a dose from scattered radiation equivalent to the dose of 1 chest radiograph.
  - Family members may stay with the patient and are required to wear a radiation badge and ring for monitoring.
  - The patient and room are monitored daily for RT safety.

External Beam RT

Localization, Immobilization, and Simulation

- ▪ Positioning: supine with head support.
- ▪ Immobilization: a device such as a thermoplast face mask is essential.
- ▪ Simulation: a CT simulation should be performed for 3D planning.

Target Volumes and Dose

- CTV: the globe or the entire retina and vitreous with lens sparing
- Dose
  - Typical does is 45 Gy/1.8 Gy/fx.
  - A dose of 36 Gy has been used alone with good local control. Some may consider this dose adjuvantly after chemotherapy or enucleation.
  - Hypofractionation has been used but is generally not recommended because of a higher risk of late effects.

Treatment Planning

- Three-dimensional imaging should be used to delineate the target and the normal tissue volumes.
  - Target should include the entire retina, and 5 to 8 mm of proximal optic nerve.
  - Organs at risk include the contralateral eye and chiasm, pituitary, brainstem, teeth, and upper cervical spine.
  - Planning goals: tumor volume is treated with the 98% line and the orbit is included in the 50% isodose line, with the organs at risk receiving less dose.
- Beam arrangement
  - Historically, orthovoltage was used with a nasal and temporal field used to spare the lens.
  - Three-dimensional and IMRT techniques (using 3-8 beams) are considered superior to the traditional D-shaped field.
  - Stereotactic radiosurgery and proton therapy are also being investigated.

PRIMITIVE NEUROECTODERMAL TUMORS

RT Indications

- This family of tumors is also known as embryonal tumors or primitive neuroectodermal tumors (PNETs), and the most common include medulloblastoma, supratentorial PNETs, and atypical teratoid rhabdoid tumors.
- Treatment for these tumors typically includes maximal surgical resection followed by chemotherapy and craniospinal EBRT.

Localization, Immobilization, and Simulation

- Positioning: prone or supine position.
  - Extend the neck to avoid divergence of the spinal field into the oral cavity. The head should be supported by a rest and positioned relative to the body to minimize cervical spine curvature and skin folds.

- Arms at the sides with the shoulders lowered to allow junction shifting.
  - Prone
    - Advantages: allows direct visual confirmation of field junctions and good alignment of the spine.
    - Disadvantages: uncomfortable, technically difficult to reproduce, and does not allow for easy intubation with anesthesia.
  - Supine
    - Advantages: comfortable, easier to reproduce, allows for intubation.
    - Disadvantages: inability to visualize bony landmarks for visual set-up confirmation (eg, visual verification of skin gap for field match).
- Immobilization: custom mold or vac-lock bag should be used for reproducible set-up, with the goal of a straight spine. Thermoplast head mask should be used to immobilize the head.
- Localization: the patient is scanned (3-5–mm slices) from the vertex to the mid-femurs. The isocenter is placed in the brain field, and triangulation points are marked on the mask. The patient is also marked at the upper thorax and pelvis for alignment.
- Simulation: computed tomography simulation is recommended to obtain 3D volumetric information of target and critical normal tissues.

Treatment Planning

- Two-dimensional field arrangement: planning begins with simulation of the spinal field first.
  - Spine: PA field from C4-7 interspace to 1 cm beyond thecal sac (visualized on sagittal MRI), extending laterally to cover transverse spinal processes
    - Controversy regarding the caudal end of the field: some question if it needs to be widened by up to 1.8 cm to encompass the increasing distance between nerve root exits as they move inferiorly down the spine, making coverage of the SI joints not necessary.
  - The lowest cervical interspace possible is used for the superior edge of the field to accommodate subsequent "feathering" of the junction.
  - If unable to encompass the entire span with a single field, 2 fields may be used with a junction gap calculated with the following equation to match fields at a specified depth and avoid convergence of beams too superficially (Figure 12.7a):

$$Separation = \frac{1}{2}\left(\frac{L * Depth}{SSD} \right)$$

Separation = gap length at skin surface
L = length of the PA spinal field

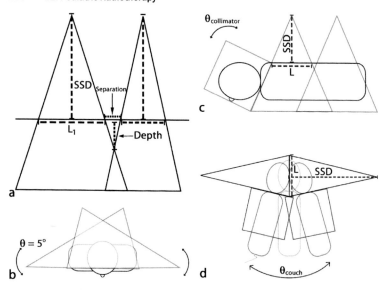

FIGURE 12.7 Depiction of cranial spinal set-up. (a) Similar triangles used for gap calculation. (b) Gantry rotation used to avoid divergence through the contralateral lens. (c) Lateral view demonstrating collimator rotation to match the divergence of the superior spine field. (d) Superior view demonstrating the table kick used to avoid the divergence of the whole-brain field into the spinal field.

Depth = depth at which the field edges superimpose
SSD = source surface distance of the PA spinal field

- Whole-brain field: German Helmet technique (see Chapter 13, WBRT) with 5° posterior tilt to spare the contralateral lens (Figure 12.7b). Blocks are designed to ensure adequate coverage of the cribriform plate and middle cranial fossa (typically 1-cm margin). If using fluoroscopic simulation, an arrow is used to mark the right bony canthus and a marker on left bony canthus.
- The collimator is rotated to match the divergence of the superior border of the spine field with the inferior border of cranial fields (Figure 12.7c).

$$\theta_{co\lim ator} = \tan^{-1}\left(\frac{1}{2} * \frac{L}{SSD} \right)$$

θ = angle of collimator rotation
L = length of the PA spinal field
SSD = source surface distance of the PA spinal field

- Divergence between the brain and spinal field is accounted for by rotating the couch toward the gantry to match the superior border of the spine field with the inferior border of cranial fields along the R-L axis (Figure 12.7d).

$$\theta_{couch} = \tan^{-1}\left(\frac{1}{2} * \frac{L}{SAD} \right)$$

θ = angle of couch kick
L = length of the lateral cranial fields
SAD = source axis distance of the lateral cranial fields

- Field matches: with the use of collimator rotation and an independent jaw technique, the cranial and spinal fields may be directly abutted (light fields). Many radiation oncologists prefer a gap between the cranial and spinal light fields; thus, a gap of 0.5 cm is allowed on most protocols. The match line should be moved superiorly by 0.5 to 1 cm after each 8 to 9 Gy (usually done once per week). Also, a penumbra broadening "match line wedge" or a dynamic wedge may be used to minimize inhomogeneity.

- 3D field arrangement: conformal treatment planning with CT simulation if available is preferred for beams-eye-view. Field arrangement and target coverage is similar to 2-dimensional planning, but calculations are not required, as collimation and table rotations are determined with the treatment planning software. Intensity-modulated radiation therapy treatment planning offers dosimetric advantages over traditional 3D-CRT in both dose homogeneity and normal tissue sparing.

Target volumes and Dose

- GTV: gross residual tumor and/or the walls of the resection cavity at the primary site from the initial and postoperative/preoperative RT imaging.
- CTV: GTV with an added margin to cover subclinical microscopic disease that is anatomically confined (ie, the CTV is limited to the confines of the bony calvarium and tentorium). There are several CTVs to take into account.
  - CTV whole brain: extends anteriorly to include the entire frontal lobe and cribriform plate. Inferiorly, the CTV1 should be at least 0.5 cm below the base of the skull at the foramen magnum.
  - CTV spine: entire cord and thecal sac. To extend laterally to cover the recesses of the entire vertebral bodies, with at least a 1-cm margin on

either side. The superior border will be the junction with the whole-brain field. The inferior border will be 2 cm below the termination of the subdural space.

- CTV posterior fossa boost: inferiorly from C1 vertebral canal through the foramen magnum, laterally to the bony walls of the occiput and temporal bones and superiorly to the tentorium cerebelli.
- PTV: in order to account for the daily setup error, the additional margin defining the PTV may range from 0.3 to 1.0 cm.

TABLE 12.7 Primitive Neuroectodermal Tumors: Organs at Risk

Structure	Dose Limit/Special Considerations
Supratentorial brain (left and right)	Avoid hot spots.
Cochlea (left and right)	32 Gy/(better visualized on CT bone window)
Hypothalamus	45 Gy/(better visualized on MRI if available)
Pituitary	45 Gy
Eyes (left and right)	50 Gy
Lens (left and right)	7 Gy
Optic nerves (left and right)	50 Gy (may go up to 59.4 Gy if necessary)
Optic chiasm	50 Gy (may go up to 59.4 Gy if necessary)
Spinal cord	50 Gy (No more than 50% of the cervical spinal cord between C1 and C2 should receive more than 54 Gy).
Cribriform plate	Better visualization and decreased error in localization with CT simulation. Important to ensure it is included in the whole brain field.
Ovaries	Be aware of dose to this structure and consider transposition or half beam blocking the inferior spinal field.
Thyroid	Try to avoid matching through this structure.

Abbreviations: CT, computed tomography.

- Dose prescription
  - Average-risk medulloblastoma: CSI to 23.4 Gy/1.8 Gy/fx followed by posterior fossa boost to 54 Gy/1.8 Gy/fx.
  - High-risk medulloblastoma and supratentorial PNET: CSI to 36 Gy/1.8 Gy/fx followed by posterior fossa boost of 18 Gy/1.8 Gy/fx to 54 Gy.
- Organs at risk (Table 12.7).
- Secondary image sets: fusion of preoperative and postoperative MRI image sets to planning CT scan should be performed. These complimentary imaging modalities assist in delineating target and critical structures as detailed above.

CRANIOPHARYNGIOMA

Radiotherapy Indications

- Radiotherapy is not indicated after gross total resection.
- Adjuvant radiotherapy is indicated after subtotal resection.
- Immediate postoperative radiotherapy provides better outcomes than does EBRT at time of recurrence.
- Radioactive colloid may be used for primary or recurrent large cystic tumors.

Localization, Immobilization, and Simulation

- Positioning: the patient should be in supine position with arms at the sides or across the chest.
- Localization: use operative reports and preoperative and postoperative MRI to delineate operative bed and/or residual disease.
- Immobilization: aquaplast face mask.
- Simulation: a CT simulation should be performed for 3D planning.

Target Volumes and Dose

- GTV: postoperative residual disease and deflated cyst as identified on MRI.
- CTV: GTV + 1- to 2-cm margin.
- Other investigative approaches have included a CTV = GTV + 5 mm and PTV = CTV + 3 mm when using imaging guidance with weekly MRI. Imaging during treatment is recommended as the cysts may grow beyond the field during treatment.
- Dose
  - 54 to 55.8 Gy/1.8 Gy/fx
  - 11 to 12 Gy in 1 fx prescribed to the 50% IDL may be considered for SRS.

TABLE 12.8 Craniopharyngioma: Critical structures

Organ	Dose Constraint (Whole or Partial Organ), Gy
Retina	45
Lens	10
Optic nerve	50
Optic chiasm	50
Brainstem	1/3, 60; 2/3, 53; 3/3, 50
Pituitary	45
Temporal lobes	1/3, 60; 2/3, 503; 3/3, 45

- Intracavitary radionuclide dose is 200 Gy to cyst wall with ^{32}P or ^{90}Y (ß emitters).
- Critical structures (Table 12.8)

Treatment Planning

- Three-dimensional imaging should be used to delineate the target and the normal tissue volumes.
- Single fraction stereotactic radiosurgery can be considered in the postoperative or recurrent setting when the tumor is 5 or more mm away from the optic chiasm.

13 Palliative Radiotherapy

Andrew D. Vassil and Gregory M. M. Videtic

GENERAL PRINCIPLES

- Palliative radiotherapy balances improving or maintaining symptom control while minimizing therapy-related adverse effects.
- Patient's performance status, physical limitations, natural disease history, and previous therapies should all be considered when designing an appropriate radiation course.
- Custom immobilization techniques, hypofractionation, brachytherapy, IMRT, intracranial SRS, SBRT, and radiopharmaceuticals may be considered when individualizing therapy.

Localization, Immobilization, and Simulation

- Positioning: assessing a patient during consultation can facilitate identifying the most comfortable and reproducible position for simulation that achieves acceptable beam arrangements (Figure 13.1a and b). Soft materials on the tabletop, such as lamb's wool, may be used to improve patient comfort.
- Immobilization: minimally restrictive devices, such as tape and straps, and more rigid devices, such as thermoplastic mesh or vacuum-locking bags, allow for easily customizable immobilization.
  - PTV margins should take the degree of immobilization into account.
  - Angled knee sponges and banding of feet aid in reproducing setup.

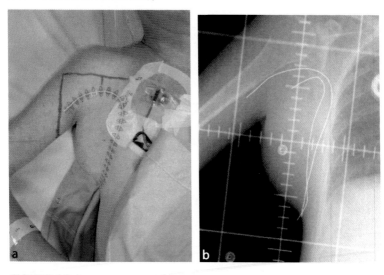

FIGURE 13.1 Patient with pain caused by right axilla metastases from melanoma. Simulation with patient supine, on soft sheep's wool table cover, arms akimbo (a). AP port showing the painful area delineated with radio-opaque wire taped to the patient's skin (b).

- SBRT requires a high degree of immobilization, typically using items such as thermoplastic molds, vacuum-locking bags, infrared localization, and intrafraction orthogonal radiograph position confirmation.
- Medication: pretreatment with analgesic and antiemetics can improve comfort during simulations and treatment.
- Localization: radiopaque markers may aid in correlating pain with simulation images (Figure 13.1 a and b).
  - Fluoroscopic or CT simulation is typically used.
  - Information from operative reports, MRI and PET studies may be incorporated to aid in target localization.
- Isocenter: for photon simulation isocenter is placed at least at D_{max} depth from the surface and typically in a central or deeper location. For electron simulation, the isocenter is placed at the skin surface.

Target Volumes and Organs of Interest Definition

- Target volumes and normal structures: ICRU guidelines should inform target delineation but may not be as strictly applied, as mandated by the patient's specific clinical needs.

Treatment Planning

- Dose prescription: a depth or location (eg, isocenter or midplane) for dose prescription allows for rapid, simple treatment planning.
- 3DCRT: when clinically necessary to reduce high doses to nontarget tissues. Oblique field angles may help avoid spinal cord and other sensitive tissues.
- IMRT: intensity-modulated radiation therapy may be favored in the setting of retreatment, for nontarget tissue sparing in selected cases, but usually comes at the expense of longer treatment times.
- Multifield and arc-beam SBRT: high conformality with dose escalation may be favored in the setting of retreatment or specific clinical scenarios.
- Electron fields: electrons are well suited to treatment of superficial lesions.
  - Choice of electron energy relates to field size and desired prescription isodose line.
  - Templates for electron cone inserts may be generated during the examination of a patient or through the use of simulation images.
  - Custom electron cone inserts may then be made and port films acquired as part of the simulation process.
- Critical structures: regions for dose limitation depend on target location.
- Beam energies: depends on target geometry and relation to surrounding structures
- Heterogeneity correction: not conventionally used
- Field matching: gantry and table rotation, and using a half-beam block can help match fields for patients undergoing a radiation course near a previously treated field or in anticipation of matching the fields in the future.

BONE METASTASES

Indications

- Techniques used to treat pain or disability from bone metastases typically use standard photon or electron external beam radiotherapy.
- Prophylactic irradiation of metastases may prevent fractures in high-risk areas, typically at the acetabulum and proximal femur.
- Hemibody radiation therapy and radiopharmaceuticals may be considered for widespread symptomatic disease.

Localization, Immobilization, and Simulation

- Positioning: comfort, reproducibility, and ease of setup favored.
  - Supine positioning is used for most situations.

- ■ Arms often at the sides but raised above the head typically when treating thoracic metastases.
- ■ Angled devices that elevate the chest may be used for patients with respiratory difficulties.
- Localization: delineating painful areas with radiopaque markers taped to the skin can help ensure that clinically involved regions are encompassed by the radiation field.
- Immobilization: for treatments of extremities, immobilization of the joint distal to the region of interest (with a vacuum-locking bag) aids in reproducing setup.
- Gantry and table rotation may be used to minimize divergence, particularly for rib lesions to avoid unnecessary lung radiation.

Target Volumes and Organs of Interest Definition

- Lesions correlating with painful areas delineated at the time of simulation are encompassed in the treatment volume.
- Radiolucency seen with lytic lesions; radiopacity is seen with blastic lesions, and areas of fracture are targeted. Regions of FDG-PET avidity and marrow infiltration/cortical destruction seen on MRI may also be included.
- Pelvic metastasis are often treated in a manner that will allow field matching if additional treatment is needed. This is accomplished by using landmarks such as the sacroiliac joint, pubic symphysis, and greater trochanter to be used as points of reference if future treatment is necessary (Figure 13.2).
- For spine metastases, target volumes that include 1 vertebral body above and below areas felt to be causing symptoms are targeted.
- After medullary fixation, the whole surgical field, all hardware, and methylmethacrylate stabilizing the bone are considered at risk for recurrence and are encompassed in the radiation field.

Treatment Planning

- Field arrangements: field arrangement depends on the region to be treated and the physical limitations of the patient and matching positioning. Examples of typical field arrangements include the following:
  - ■ AP/PA (extremities, sacrum, and pelvis)
  - ■ PA (lumbar, thoracic spine)
  - ■ En face electron (skull, scapula, sternum, rib, and clavicle)
  - ■ Lateral and oblique parallel opposed (cervical spine and rib)
  - ■ Wedged pairs (rib and superficial lesions)

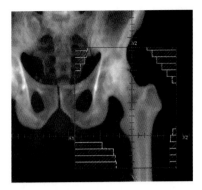

FIGURE 13.2 Patient with pain caused by a left femoral head/neck metastasis from prostate cancer. This patient previously received 70 Gy prostate bed salvage radiotherapy. AP portal targeting femoral head/neck.

Dose/Fractionation

- The patient's performance status, natural history of the patient's disease, previous therapies, and inherent sensitivity of a given histology should all be considered when determining a radiation dose and fractionation.
  - A dose of 8 Gy delivered in a single fx with 6- to 10-MV photons or electrons is effective in most situations. A dose of 20 to 30 Gy delivered in 5 to 10 fx may also be considered.
  - A dose of 30 Gy delivered in 10 fx is safe and typically given 10 to 14 days after surgical procedures such as spinal decompression and medullary fixation.
- Re-irradiation: treating beyond normal tissue tolerance should be avoided, unless mandated by the patient's need. Consider alternative radiotherapy techniques.
- Hemibody radiation: This technique is useful for patients with widespread painful bone metastases.
  - Fields are divided at the umbilicus or L4/L5 with an extended SSD with 6- to 10-MV photons.
  - Transmission lung blocks limit midline lung dose to 6 to 7 Gy.
  - 6 Gy delivered to the upper body and 8 Gy delivered to the lower body in 1 fx
  - Alternatively, 15 Gy in 5 fx, 20-30 Gy in 8-10 fx given 3 fx per week
  - The other half of the body is treated 6 to 8 weeks later.

- Radiopharmaceuticals: β-particle emitting radiopharmaceuticals typically used.
  - Strontium-89 and Samarium-153 are most common.
  - These incorporate into bone hydroxyapatite.
  - Radiopharmaceuticals may be considered for patients with multiple blastic lesions from breast and prostate cancer.

SBRT FOR SPINE METASTASES

Introduction

- Typically used for patients with high performance status, low volume of disease, and radiobiologically resistant disease, with symptomatic disease recurrence in a previous radiation field.
- Potential advantages of SBRT: bone marrow preservation by treating limited volumes, convenience of fewer patient visits compared with fractionated therapy, less interference with ongoing chemotherapy treatments, use as a decompressive therapy for those with epidural compression, and noninvasive alternative to surgery.
- Disadvantages of SBRT: cost, complexity, patient tolerability, delay in time to initiation of treatment, field size limitations, duration of radiation delivery, necessary specialized equipment, and benefits over conventional radiotherapy remain to demonstrated.
- The following is based in part on the RTOG 0631 protocol.

Localization, Immobilization, and Simulation

- Positioning: due to the prolonged duration of treatment fractions, a comfortable supine position must be found.
- Localization: systems that relate patient position to the table and isocenter are used.
  - A frame with a stereotactic localization coordinate system may be used.
  - Depending on the method of image guidance to be used at the time of treatment, fiducial markers (eg, infrared reflective) may be placed on the frame and patient.
- Immobilization: rigid immobilization systems are used because of the necessary setup precision.
  - Custom devices providing multiple points of contact are used.
  - Examples include a vacuum-locking bag or thermoplastic mask for cervical spine treatments.
- Thin slice simulation CT (typically 2 mm) is coregistered with high-resolution magnetic resonance images (T1 with gadolinium contrast and T2 sequences) to aid in target delineation.

- IGRT: internal landmarks (eg, bone and fiducial implants) verifying positioning should be less than 2 mm from the simulation position. IGRT devices to verify patient position may involve orthogonal imaging, CBCT, electronic portal imaging devices, and CT-on-rails systems.

Target Volumes and Organs of Interest Definition

- Definition of the PTV
  - Involved vertebral body, pedicles, and gross disease including paraspinal masses (Figure 13.3).
  - Transverse processes, lamina, and spinus process are included when the disease is located in posterior vertebral elements.
  - A space 3 mm or greater space between the spinal cord and PTV should be present.
  - Paraspinal mass should be 5 cm or less.
- Critical structures
  - Spinal cord: delineated on MRI; 5 to 6 mm superior and inferior to the level of the CTV, depending on CT slice thickness.
  - Normal organs should also be delineated when these structures are in the beam path.

Treatment Planning

- Photon energy: typically, 6-MV photons are used, given the decreased penumbra and reduced exit dose relative to higher energy photons.

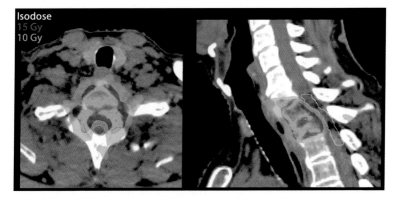

FIGURE 13.3 Patient with vertebral body metastases previously irradiated with conventional technique. PTV (blue line) and spinal cord (yellow line) delineated on axial and sagittal planes; 16 Gy (purple) and 10 Gy (green) isodose "clouds". Nonopposed, coplanar beams with 6-MV photons used.

- Dose rate: to limit treatment time, 800 monitor units/minute or higher is desired.
- Beam arrangement: multiple posterior nonopposed coplanar beams or posterior arc beam fields with the beam isocenter at the center of the PTV. Noncoplanar beams and IMRT may be used for irregularly shaped targets.
- Prescription point: prescription is typically to the 80% to 90% IDL. A dose greater than 105% of the prescription dose should not be outside of the PTV.
- Normal tissue limits: 10% of the spinal cord (5-6 mm above and below the PTV) should be limited to receive 10 Gy. Less than 0.35 cc of the spinal cord should receive 10 Gy. Reconstructions with isodose displayed should be reviewed to ensure that no region is receiving a higher than acceptable dose, particularly the spinal cord. Refer to the RTOG 0631 protocol for dose restriction guidelines.

Dose/Fractionation

- For de novo treatments, 16 Gy is prescribed to include at least 90% of the PTV.
- When treating a volume within a previously irradiated field, 14 Gy is used.

BRAIN METASTASES—WBRT

Introduction

- WBRT is used as a single modality or in conjunction with surgery, SRS, and chemotherapy.
- A slightly larger field ("German helmet") is also used, especially when there is a concern for leptomeningeal spread of disease or with posterior fossa lesions.

Localization, Immobilization, and Simulation

- Positioning: the patient is positioned supine with the head in a neutral position. Radiopaque markers are at the fleshy canthus bilaterally.
- Localization: head rotation is corrected before making the immobilization mask by viewing the position of the laser lines on structures such as the nose and auditory canal. Fluoroscopy or scout image may be taken to confirm head position.
- Immobilization: a thermoplastic mask is made.
- Lateral radiographs or CT images are acquired.

Target Volumes and Organs of Interest Definition

- Definition of the PTV
    - Clinical setup of the field is done to include the entire brain; if CT planning is used, review of axial images can help ensure that the entire brain is included and dose to nontarget structures is minimized.
    - Attention is paid to ensure adequate margin on the cribriform plate and temporal lobes.
    - The posterior half of the orbits are included in a German helmet field, in an effort to include all meningeal surface (Figure 13.4b and d).
- Critical structures
    - Normal tissues such as the lenses, posterior oropharynx, and posterior neck soft tissues may be avoided by blocking with primary collimator rotation, 5–HVL layer cerrobend blocks, or multileaf collimators.

Treatment Planning

- Photon energy: typically, 6-MV photons are used.
- Beam arrangement: opposed lateral fields, with the isocenter placed at midplane; for German helmet plans, a 5° gantry rotation is used to create anteriorly nondivergent fields that avoid treating the lenses (Figure 13.4b and d).
- Fields
    - Standard WBRT fields: the collimator is rotated to block the anterior orbit and tissues anterior to the skull base; a 1-cm border anterior to the skull base is typically adequate to ensure coverage of the temporal lobe (Figure 13.4a).
    - German helmet field: a 5° posterior gantry rotation minimizes divergence into the lens. The collimator is kept at 90°, the C2-3 interspace is used for the inferior boarder (Figure 13.4b).
    - The field is opened to provide margin superiorly and posteriorly at least 1 cm beyond the skull (ie, "flash").
    - Blocking at the C1-2 interspace may be used for whole-brain fields for the purpose of potentially matching fields in the future.

Dose/Fractionation

- No fractionation schedule is superior to another based on randomized studies, and RT prescription often reflects patient performance and institutional practice.
- In the United States, 30 Gy/3 Gy/fx is commonly used and is also used after surgical resection of metastases.
- Typically, 37.5 Gy/2.5 Gy/fx is used for patients who will or have received SRS (1).

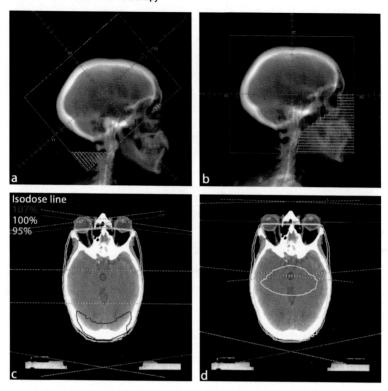

FIGURE 13.4 Right lateral standard WBRT field (a) and German helmet field (b). Isodose distribution displaying the 100% (yellow), 107% (red), and 95% (blue) isodose lines for WBRT (c) and German helmet fields (d).

- 20 Gy/5 Gy/fx: often for patients with poor performance status and active extracranial disease
- 20 Gy/2 Gy/fx: in the setting of repeat WBRT after a patient has previously received 25 to 37.5 Gy
- Appropriateness criteria have been produced by the American College of Radiology (2).

BRAIN METASTASES—SRS

Introduction

- SRS uses multiple beam paths to provide high doses of radiation with rapid dose fall-off for intracranial metastatic lesions typically 40 mm or less in maximum dimension.

- SRS requires extremely precise immobilization, imaging, and radiation delivery.
    - Delivery systems: Gamma-knife (GK, Elekta, Stockholm, Sweden) radiosurgery system; Cyberknife (Accuray, Sunnyvale, CA); modified traditional linear accelerator (eg, Novalis, Palo Alto, CA).

Localization, Immobilization, and Simulation

- Immobilization: frame-based and "frameless" techniques are used
    - A rigid metal frame is attached to the skull with 4 screws. The frame provides immobilization, stereotactic localization systems attach to the frame.
    - Attention is paid to the location of the targets in reference to the frame position, to avoid placing the frame directly over the target lesion(s).
    - Frameless immobilization uses a thermoplastic mask, infrared fiducial markers, and orthogonal radiograph guidance during radiation delivery.
- Localization: high-resolution CT and MRI studies (1-mm slice thickness) are conducted with the patient supine and the frame locked to the imaging table.
    - Image sets are coregistered using the stereotactic fiducial coordinate system attached to the frame (Figure 13.5a).
    - A skull scaling device is used to make external head contour measurements for GK planning to assess beam path length in tissue. This is particularly useful when the entire head is not imaged, and surface data are not available.
    - Other treatment planning systems may use the head contour delineated from simulation CT.
- Immobilization: this frame attaches to the treatment table, immobilizing the patient's head.

Target Volumes and Organs of Interest Definition

- Definition of the PTV
    - Metastatic lesions are delineated on MRI coregistered to simulation CT.
    - Target volumes should be at least 5 mm away from the optic chiasm and nerves.
- Critical structures
    - The optic chiasm is delineated on MRI coregistered to CT; coronal views aid in identifying the optic chiasm.

Treatment Planning

- GK and Cyberknife systems use spherical points of radiation dose ("shots" for GK, "nodes" for Cyberknife) generated by fixed circular collimators.

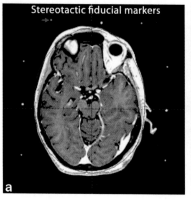
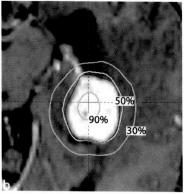

FIGURE 13.5 Stereotactic coordinate system used for image registration (a); typical isodose distribution in a GK plan encompassing metastatic lesion with the 50% IDL (b).

The "shots" or "nodes" can be abutted with forward planning to generate irregularly shaped isodose distributions.

- The GK Perfexion system uses multiple focused "sectors" of varying collimator sizes to generate irregularly shaped isodose distributions.
- Cyberknife systems use fixed circular collimators and delivers "nodes" from multiple gantry positions with the use of a linear accelerator mounted on a robotic arm. A "step-and-shoot" technique is used; that is, radiation is not delivered while the robotic arm is moving.
- Linear accelerator-based treatment typically uses 6 to 8 arced photon fields. Varying the fixed circular collimator ("cone") size or MLC shape ("dynamic arc"), number and position of isocenters, number of arcs, arc angle, degree of arc rotation, and weight of each arc can help shape the isodose distribution to conform to the target. To improve dose conformity to the target, IMRT may be used.
- After planning is complete, DVH and isodose distributions on all images should be reviewed to ensure that areas of unacceptably high dose are not falling on critical normal structures, such as the optic chiasm.
- Dose is prescribed in a manner such that the 50% IDL encompasses that target lesion for GK systems (Figure 13.5b); the 80% isodose line is used for linear accelerator-based systems. This is the "median marginal dose," that is, the median dose at the target margin.
- Conformity index is the prescribed isodose volume divided by the target volume and should be have a value between 1 and 2.

- Homogeneity index is the maximum dose divided by the prescribed dose and should be a value less than 2.

Dose/Fractionation

- Per RTOG 90-05, a single fx of 24 Gy for lesions 2 cm or less, 18 Gy for 2.1 to 3.0 cm, and 15 Gy for 3.1 to 4.0 cm are used.

MALIGNANT OBSTRUCTIONS AND BLEEDING

Introduction

- Debilitating and life-threatening events can be caused by intrinsic and extrinsic airway obstruction, superior vena cava (SVC) compression, and esophageal compression and bleeding.
- EBRT can provide durable symptom relief and may be combined with other therapies.
- Brachytherapy may also provide durable relief but should not be combined with concurrent chemotherapy.

Localization, Immobilization, and Simulation

- Positioning: in most situations, patients are simulated supine with arms above the head.
  - In cases of severe airway and SVC obstruction, patients may be more comfortable on an angled board to elevate the thorax.
  - An upright, seated position can be used for patients who cannot tolerate a supine position.
- Localization: oral contrast (such as gastrograffin) helps identify esophageal obstruction and may identify tracheoesophageal fistula.
  - Tracheoesophageal fistula is not a contraindication for EBRT; however, brachytherapy is believed to be unsafe in this setting.
  - Endoscopic placement of a 6- to 10-mm diameter catheter is done for brachytherapy procedures. Distance and active length measurements are made at the time of catheter placement and verified at time of simulation. Surgical clips may be placed endoscopically to delineate the extent of disease in cases of esophageal obstruction.
- Immobilization: rigid immobilization is typically not needed. For patients in a seated position, a rigid back rest is used for consistent setup. For brachytherapy, the catheter is marked at the level of the incisors and taped to the patient's face to keep it from migrating.
- CT simulation is preferred over fluoroscopic simulation to better visualize the extent of disease.

Target Volumes and Organs of Interest Definition

- Definition of the PTV
  - Gross disease (GTV) causing obstruction should be included with a 1.5- to 2-cm combined CTV/PTV expansion.
- Critical structures
  - Normal organs should also be delineated when these structures are in the beam path.

Treatment Planning

- EBRT: typically, 6-MV photons are used with anteroposterior/PA fields for most sites.
- Brachytherapy: 3D planning is preferred (Figure 13.6).
  - Active length for brachytherapy is determined by the length of disease seen at endoscopy and on simulation CT.
  - Source dwell time optimization may be used to expand coverage at the distal portions of the active length.
  - Active length should be 10 cm or less.

Dose/Fractionation

- For esophageal brachytherapy, 10 to 14 Gy HDR in 2 fx 1 week apart is prescribed at a 1-cm radius from the midsource position. Also, LDR may be used to deliver 20 to 25 Gy in a single fx at 0.4 to 1 Gy/h (3).
- For endobronchial brachytherapy, 15 Gy HDR prescribed in a similar fractionation and depth as esophageal brachytherapy may be used.
- EBRT dosing for situations of bleeding, bronchial and SVC obstruction: include hypofractioned regiments such as 17 Gy/8.5 Gy/fx separated by 1 week or 20 to 30 Gy/3 to 4 Gy/fx.
- EBRT dosing for esophageal obstruction is 30 Gy/3 Gy/fx; more protracted radiation courses and/or combined chemotherapy reflect patient status and clinical judgment.

SKIN AND SOFT TISSUE METASTASES

Introduction

- Techniques for treating soft tissue metastasis include photon or electron fields and may involve SBRT.
- Hyperthermia may serve as an adjunctive therapy in situations of re-irradiation of superficial soft tissues such as a chest wall recurrence.
- Radioactive yttrium-90 microspheres may be considered for treatment of liver metastases.

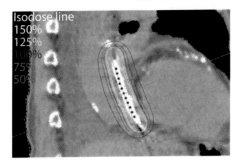

FIGURE 13.6 Patient with bleeding from an esophageal cancer now being treated with brachytherapy. Isodose distribution for prescription normalized to a depth of 0.5 cm. Brachytherapy source dwell positions are noted with red dots.

Localization, Immobilization, and Simulation

- Head and neck skin and nodal metastasis: position the patient supine with head extended and shoulders down; a thermoplastic mask is made and the patient is imaged from vertex to carina or inferior extent of disease (eg, mediastinal disease). Bolus may be applied under the mask; thus, the mask will aid in keeping bolus material in place during treatment.

- Pancoast syndromes: position the patient supine, head rotated contralateral to the disease, arms above the head or at side; image from mastoid tip to inferior aspect of thorax (to ensure imaging of entire lung tissue).

- Pulmonary and mediastinal metastasis: position the patient supine with arms above the head or at the side; image from midneck to inferior aspect of thorax (to ensure imaging of entire lung tissue). In cases of oligometastatic pulmonary disease, SBRT may be considered.

- Liver metastases: position the patient supine with arms above the head; image from thoracic inlet to iliac crests; 4D-CT may be considered in an effort to reduce PTV margins, particularly for patients who have received prior radiation therapy near the target region. For oligometastatic disease, SBRT may be considered.

- Pelvic malignancies: the patient is positioned supine with arms across the chest; image from the level of the L1 vertebral body to the lesser trochanter.

- Skin metastases: bolus material, typically 1 cm thick, may be custom cut to encompass volumes delineated by radiopaque marker with additional 2- to 3-cm margin. Simulation imaging may be conducted with bolus over the region to be treated; alternatively, bolus material may be designed using the treatment planning software, then custom cut.

- CT simulation is generally preferred.

Target Volumes and Organs of Interest Definition

- Definition of the PTV
  - Gross disease (GTV) identified on CT simulation causing obstruction and palpable disease should be included with a 1.5- to 2-cm combined CTV/PTV expansion.
  - Skin, head, and neck: areas clinically involved as identified by patient history, physical examination, and imaging are delineated at the time of simulation. Regional lymphatics may be included in the treatment field depending on histology and factors such as performance status and prior radiation fields.
- Critical structures
  - Normal structures surrounding the PTV (eg, parotid glands, spinal cord, esophagus, normal lung tissue, kidneys, and liver) should be delineated and considered in treatment planning.

Treatment Planning

- Generally, 3D planning with 6- to 10-MV photons or electrons of energy to encompass PTV within the 80% to 100% IDL is used.
- Electron templates may be designed without simulation imaging for well-defined, palpable, superficial lesions that have recently been characterized by volumetric staging studies, such as CT. Target areas may be marked on the patient's skin with ink, a transparent film is overlaid and the area is traced. An electron cone insert is made from the traced area and appropriate electron energy is chosen based on desired target dimensions.

Dose/Fractionation

- In most situations, for patients with skin or soft tissue metastases, 20 to 30 Gy/3 to 4 Gy/fx can be used.
- Alternatives include
  - Melanoma and renal cell carcinoma: 5 Gy/fx, twice weekly to a total dose of 30 Gy
  - Liver metastases (whole or partial liver): 10 Gy delivered in 2 fx separated by 6 to 24 hours (4)
  - Adrenal metastases: 30 Gy/2.5 to 3 Gy/fx
  - Splenomegally from leukemia: 5 to 10 Gy delivered in 1-Gy fx given 3 times a week
  - Pelvic malignancies: 10 Gy in 1 fx, may be repeated after 4 weeks
  - Skin metastases: 8 Gy in 1 fx

REFERENCES

1. Andrews DW, Scott CB, Sperduto PW, et al. Whole brain radiation therapy with or without stereotactic radiosurgery boost for patients with one to three brain metastases: phase III results of the RTOG 9508 randomised trial. *Lancet.* 2004;363:1665–1672.

2. Videtic GM, Gaspar LE, Aref AM, et al. American College of Radiology appropriateness criteria on multiple brain metastases. *Int J Radiat Oncol Biol Phys.* 2009;75:961–965.

3. Gaspar LE, Nag S, Herskovic A, Mantravadi R, Speiser B. American Brachytherapy Society (ABS) consensus guidelines for brachytherapy of esophageal cancer. Clinical Research Committee, American Brachytherapy Society, Philadelphia, PA. *Int J Radiat Oncol Biol Phys.* 1997;38:127–132.

4. Bydder S, Spry NA, Christie DR, et al. A prospective trial of short-fractionation radiotherapy for the palliation of liver metastases. *Australas Radiol.* 2003;47:284–288.

Index